"I
wi
wi

"V

"I'

"I
to
- n
ju
in

"I
th

"I

"He
it tha 2100204/6 ~ 3
sets ou
completely but we can simplify, delegate, and think differently about what we
have to do. Perhaps these are the keys to staying sane... This book provides a
variety of helpful strategies."

Tami Brady DD, RM (TCM Reviews)

"It's brilliant! Funny, interesting, informative and enjoyable. Thank-you!"

Tina Kirkman, West Yorkshire UK

Published by Kirkman Raine Books, England

email: enquiries@kirkmanrainebooks.com
www.kirkmanrainebooks.com

ISBN: 978-0-9564939-0-3

Editing: Jill Bailin
Proofreading: Alison Bayne
Cover Design: Danielle Raine
Text Design: Daisy Kirkman
Text set in Garamond Regular 11pt/13.5pt.

Disclaimer
The advice in this book is intended as helpful hints towards general well-being. It is not intended as a substitute for medical or professional advice. In dealing with any medical or mental health condition, always consult a physical or mental health professional. The personal evidence contained herein is anecdotal and the author claims no relevant official qualifications other than life experience. The author accepts no responsibility for the actions of the reader as a result of reading this book. The reader is responsible for evaluating the suitability or appropriateness of the ideas herein with relation to their own life.

*This book is dedicated to...*

Women everywhere, for the invisible work they do,

&

my family - my inspiration.

# Housework
# Blues

## A SURVIVAL GUIDE

How to cope with the mental and
emotional challenge of keeping a home

Danielle Raine

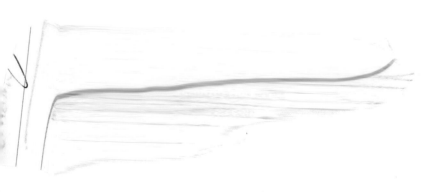

## Warning

This is not a practical housekeeping manual.

There may be the odd tip or useful gem, but the main aim of this book is not to teach you how to clean your home. My intention is to help you cope with the *unique psychological challenge* of being a modern female with a home to keep. This book is less 'how to' and more 'why bother'. These are strategies to keep you sane.

If, like me, you lack the domestic gene where housework comes naturally, or your feminist tendencies make you want to run screaming from mop and bucket, then this book is for you. It's a collection of ideas that I've stumbled across, ideas that have eased the mental burden of doing what must be done within the home.

My wish is that these simple suggestions will save you years of anguish and frustration. And I hope that these perspectives will liberate you to enjoy a beautiful home with both your sanity and relationships intact.

## A note to the naturally sceptical

You will get the greatest benefit from this book if you approach it with a very open mind.

Some of the most revolutionary insights may come from unconventional, even controversial, sources. In my search for solutions, I've studied ancient philosophies, Eastern religions, quantum physics, metaphysics, business tycoons, success gurus, NLP, spirituality, and psychology. Some of the following concepts may stretch, even counter, your currently held beliefs. But if those beliefs aren't working – what have you got to lose?

You may think an idea is poppycock, but if it gets you through the daily grind without throttling anyone - *why not go with poppycock?*

Einstein's definition of insanity:
doing the same thing over and over again
and expecting different results.

# Contents

# Intro

# How this book came to be

*When I was just a little girl...*

I asked my mother, 'What will I be? Will I be pretty? Will I be rich?'

But she didn't say, 'Que sera, sera…' She said, 'If you're planning to marry and have children, you'd better learn to like cooking and cleaning.'

So I decided on the spot that, no, I would not marry or have children because I was meant for 'better things' than the drudgery of housewifery. (Well, it was the eighties, when women could 'Have it all!'...)

This approach went swimmingly until one day, many years later, I woke up to discover that I had indeed acquired both husband and children. But that was fine, as these were a source of great joy and happiness.

Less joyful was the role I'd unwittingly landed, as House Slave.

I didn't remember *that* clause in the marriage vows. Nor any warning in the many motherhood manuals I devoured during pregnancy. Nobody warns you about all the sheer volume of domestic stuff.

So, it's possible that this book may fill that role - serving as a gentle warning to any woman about to enter the 'homemaking' phase of her life. Mostly, though, it's for women like me who are already there - bewildered, frustrated and wondering how the hell to cope.

## Housework - it does your head in.

For the majority of my married life (eleven years at the time of this writing), one phrase could sum up my attitude to housework –'It does my head in.'

It wasn't my knees that suffered, as in days of yore, or fingers, worked to the bone. In fact, it wasn't technically my head, in the physical sense, but more accurately my mind. After much anguish, guilt and soul-searching, I discovered that my resentment of domestic strife was actually a *mental issue.*

For a while I pretended it was merely a time thing. I used to say, *I never find the time to mop the floor.* Yet there would always be time to read books (often, ironically, about housework), or watch *Desperate Housewives,* or sit in cafes, perusing magazines about beautiful homes.

So the problem clearly wasn't a lack of hours in the day.

From there I declared it a lack of inclination – *I've got better things to do than dust ornaments…* et cetera… Yet, deep down, I yearned for a beautiful, clean and tidy home. I envied others who seemed to manage it. I was wracked with guilt and shame, should anyone call unexpectedly, when the house was a mess (which was any day with a 'y' in it). So, neither was it a case of indifference – not only did I care; I cared deeply.

Gradually, I suspected that the problem lay in my self-image. Being a product of the Have It All generation, perhaps it was a feminist thing? When it came to housework, my feminist tendencies were roaring, *Why should* women *do it?* But on top of this, I discovered a psychological torment (*must it be done over and over and over?*) which progressed to an existential one (*must it be done at all?*).

After much pondering (housework at least gives you plenty of time to think), the solution eventually dawned on me. I realised that the only difference between me and other women - who seemed to cope with housework and stay sane - was one of *attitude*.

## It's all in the mind

I concluded that my brain just wasn't wired to merely *get on with* the domestic stuff. It needed *valid reasons* to cope with the repetition, the injustice and the futility. And after recognising this mental aspect, it became easier to explain the emotional issues, i.e., the housework blues. After all, if your thoughts about housework are predominantly negative, they're unlikely to lead to feelings of joy, motivation or even inclination.

So I began a quest. I sought alternative ideas and new perspectives which would help me cope more positively with the task at hand. Gradually, through books, chats with friends, the internet, even overheard snippets of conversation, I came across some real gems of insight. These weren't complex theories. Quite often they were just a different way of looking at things.

But, for me, these new approaches meant the difference between sanity and running screaming from the kitchen. Or the difference between domestic bliss and the divorce court. Or the difference between family harmony and my offspring growing up to remember me as the permanently cross lady who kept a messy house.

In short, big differences. And all from just simple nuggets of wisdom. How I wished I had known these ten years ago! But failing time-travel, if I can share these ideas with others, then my battle has not been in vain.

So it's my sincere wish that you'll benefit from what I learned the hard way. I hope that the suggestions in the following pages will bring mental and emotional relief, easing the struggle that keeping a home can become. My aim is to close the gap between your current frazzled reality and the calmer, healthier, happier version of you. (She's in there somewhere.)

Also, although housework is a universal issue, the role of homemaker is a uniquely feminine one. So, even though many of these ideas will help anyone, regardless of gender, the perspective is tailored to the needs of modern women. The underlying theme is to support women in our singular role in the world, empowering us to better care for ourselves and our loved ones and also to fulfill more of our potential - beyond housework.

I believe that in this small way, by helping women survive/conquer their Housework Blues, the world may be a calmer, happier and more pleasant place. And our homes will be a good deal more enjoyable, too.

So, I hope you'll take comfort in these musings from a kindred soul. Moreover, I hope you'll find a certain peace and serenity in the answers I've discovered.

Power to your elbow (grease).

# The trouble with housework...

I hate housework. You make the beds,
you wash the dishes... and six months later
you have to start all over again.

*- Joan Rivers*

Women are capable and resilient creatures, able to multi-task, organise, plan, nurture, coordinate and generally cope with some of life's toughest demands. We can produce a human being from our bodies. When our loved ones are at risk, we're able to perform feats of superhuman strength. As a race, we're incredible!

Yet throughout the ages one thing has been the bane of womankind - *housework*. It gets us down. But what is it with housework? Why does it get to us so much? Well, from my own experience, I have identified that the Housework Blues tend to stem from one (or more) of eight particular complaints.

See if you recognize any of the grievances on the following page:

## 1. Overwhelmed

*There's too much to do.*
*I don't know where to start.*
*I never get on top of my jobs.*

## 2. Injustice

*Why should I do it all?*
*I didn't make the mess.*
*Why am I the only one doing it?*

## 3. Futility

*What's the point?*
*It'll only get dirty again.*
*It's endless.*

## 4. No Energy

*I can't be bothered.*
*I'm too tired.*
*It's too much like hard work.*

## 5. Boredom

*It's so monotonous.*
*Every day, the same chores, over and over.*
*I hate repetitive tasks.*

## 6. Inferiority

*I'm no good at this.*
*I'm so useless.*
*Other women can manage it but not me.*

## 7. Superiority

*I'm better than this.*
*It's a waste of my brain and talents.*
*Is this where I've ended up?*

## 8. Lack of Motivation

*I can't seem to get started.*
*I just don't want to do it.*
*I'd rather do something else.*

Unfortunately, these attitudes are very common - even though they can make our work unnecessarily tough. But the good news is: for all of these mindsets, there's an alternative way to view the problem. And these new perspectives, insights and ideas are the core content of this book.

The following solutions will undoubtedly bring you more success and control in the domestic realm. More importantly, though, they'll increase both your inner peace and your outer harmony. And banishing these unnecessary and unpleasant Housework Blues will have a sublime ripple effect that will benefit your whole life immeasurably.

## Intuitive solution-finding

This book has been split into eight sections, each one addressing one of the above complaints. In this way, it's easy for you to go straight to the issue you most resonate with. Identifying the problem is a vital first step towards the solution, so trust your instinct. Use your famous intuition. You may find that you are drawn to an issue which you feel is illogical or irrelevant but if you are drawn to it at all, there's a reason. Sometimes your instinct knows what you need better than your conscious mind.

It's possible that some of the tips you come across may not appeal to you immediately, and it's fine to cherry-pick your favourites. But I believe they're all worth considering and you never know where that life-changing nugget of insight may be hiding. Also, try to keep an open mind - what may not work for you today, may make total sense one day in the future.

You may also notice that some of the advice is contradictory. This is not a mistake. Not only are we humans all different, each one of us can be fickle and contrary beings. As our moods change, we'll need to alter our approach. So it pays to have an arsenal of wide-ranging perspectives to draw on.

Also, it's not necessary to memorise this information. One reading will implant these suggestions in your psyche, where they will await the opportune moment to spring forth and make your life easier and happier - the way it's meant to be.

So, consider the eight core 'issues' again. Notice how you feel as you read them, then go straight to the one that calls to you the most.

It's time to beat those Housework Blues.

The cruel irony
of housework

~

people only notice
when you don't do it.

# Section 1:

# Overwhelm

Please note, I realise that to use 'overwhelm' as a noun is grammatically incorrect. However, in the spirit of language being used to convey meaning, I am going to use it to describe 'the sense of being overwhelmed', as I believe you know what I mean...

# Where do I start?

I once read an article about a woman who loved puzzles. Nothing earth-shattering about that, but the piece had a profound effect on me. When describing her hobby, this otherwise ordinary lady said, 'Every afternoon, when I've finished all my jobs, I sit down with a cup of tea, a biscuit and my favourite puzzle book.'

Did you spot the remarkable bit?

'...finished all my jobs...'

When I read that, I was shocked. I had never known such a scenario! It was like a view into another world... a world where you can relax, happy in the knowledge that your home is clean and tidy and there is nothing to be done. (At least for a while.)

This situation had *never happened* in my life. Ever. If I found myself sitting down and relaxing (which I must admit, is something I force myself to do regularly...), it was always with the gnawing sense that I should be doing something else. The washing-up was beckoning me, or there was laundry to be hung out, or a meal to organise, a bathroom to clean, vacuuming, dusting, tidying, sorting, planning, etc, etc, etc...

It dawned on me that my overwhelming perception of housework was precisely that - *overwhelming*. It was all, literally, too much. I'd previously thought that this was just the way it was, so it was a real eye-opener to discover that some women actually get on top of the situation.

I envied that puzzle-woman, who was so accomplished that she 'got all her jobs done'. I decided that I wanted that for myself.

## The dangers of overwhelm

Once I discovered this covetable 'other way', I felt sure it must be a more pleasant - and healthful - way to live. After all, feelings of being overwhelmed don't just affect the state of your home - they also have a destructive effect on your physical and mental state. By definition, to overwhelm is to 'bury or drown beneath a huge mass, defeat completely'. A sense of being overwhelmed can trigger a downward spiral that could lead to illness and depression. In this light, then, too much housework can actually damage your health.

So, with the puzzle-lady as my role model, I set about finding solutions to my feelings of overwhelm. I decided to take back control. I refused to be beaten by the dust and dirty dishes. If there was a way to be victorious on the domestic front, I was going to find it.

Little did I know at the time that in my new-found determination, I had unwittingly fought my first battle – The Declaration of Intention.

## The power of intention.

Did you know that you can conquer your negative feelings simply by intending to do so? It's possible to eliminate fear, just by deciding not to be afraid. It can be that simple. (Not easy, but simple.) You can defuse anger, jealousy, guilt or any unpleasant emotion, just by refusing to feel it.

Such is the power of intention.

Unswerving intent has enormous power behind it and it's a power we can turn to our aid. My intention became to rise above feelings of overwhelm within my home, to no longer accept the idea that 'it' was all too much. And with that small shift of attitude, I'd taken a giant leap toward my goal. The power of this intention would prove to be a driving force in defeating overwhelm.

Despite this promising first step, however, there was still a long way to go before I could reach for the puzzle book. Determination may have been a great start, but information and knowledge were to prove vital to my success. Which is why I invite you to share the following techniques. These are useful insights and strategies that I stumbled across in my bid to conquer the domestic realm, and they have proven to be dependable allies.

So, if you too would like to know that magical feeling of being competent, capable and in control of your home, make the decision - right now - to reject overwhelm. Make that vital mental shift that you *can* and *will* be victorious!

Then you can relax for a bit as you discover how to go about it...

# Eliminate

If a thing's worth doing, it's worth doing well.

This may be true, but some things are not worth doing. (Whilst other things could be made easier or even done by someone else - more on that later...) If you feel that you simply have too much to do, you could be right. So the solution is either to accomplish more (easier said than done) or have less to do.

In the spirit of the latter, let's start by looking for any areas that can be eliminated.

## Declutter your home

First things first - are you cleaning/dusting/falling over more stuff than you need to? Could you live with fewer 'things'?

Clear or empty spaces are soothing to the mind and in cases of overwhelm, they are the Holy Grail. So, a good first step in regaining domestic control is to hold a major review of the objects that fill your home.

Life-coaches are big fans of this strategy - and with good reason. The process of simply getting rid of items you no longer want, use or need can re-energise your whole life. You create the necessary space for new possibilities and opportunities. It will also lift the mental pressure of having too many belongings. Common reactions, after a thorough purge, are sensations of lightness, optimism and relief - these are powerful antidotes to Housework Blues.

So get the de-cluttering bug. (It can actually become quite addictive). Adopt a discerning mindset. Try to gradually reduce your environment to what you need and what you love.

Even if you like to be surrounded by lots of things, just make sure they are things you enjoy. De-cluttering doesn't have to mean throwing away your beloved items or creating a stark, minimalist interior (although that would be easier to keep clean...) Go at a pace that's comfortable for you. However, do try to be honest with yourself. As you appraise your belongings, keep in mind your goal of conquering overwhelm.

For everything in your home, ask yourself, *Do I need it?* or *Do I love it?* If the answer is no to both, then ask, *Why am I cleaning it?* (or not, as the case may be...) With websites such as eBay and freecycle, it's now easier than ever to pass on unwanted items that are too good to throw away. (Although the good old car boot sale is still a potentially lucrative way to recycle your old belongings.)

A good time to have a big sort-out is before Christmas (to make room for what Santa brings!) or before birthdays, particularly children's birthdays. Whilst these biannual purges are effective, it's a habit of *regular clutter-busting* that brings lasting benefits. You will dramatically reduce not only what needs cleaning/tidying, but also the amount of time it takes to do so. There will also be a bonus side effect of boosted energy levels. It's a triple whammy! Personally, I've found decluttering to be one of the most satisfying and effective techniques to helping me feel competent and in control. (At least until I notice the laundry pile...)

Once you have rid your home of extraneous clutter, you will need to remain vigilant, to make sure it doesn't creep back in. When shopping for new items, think twice about what you choose to give house-space (and subsequently brain-space). You may love that new *objet d'art*, but are you going to love cleaning it? (Or, perhaps more likely, will you love looking at it covered in dust/fingerprints/cereal/all of the above?)

> Have nothing in your house that you do not know to be useful, or believe to be beautiful.
>
> *William Morris*

So, if the clutter-free way appeals to you, you would do yourself, your family and your home a valuable service by learning the tricks and techniques. There are many inspiring and informative resources available which deal with de-cluttering in more depth. Two of my personal favourite books are: *Cut the Clutter* by Cynthia Townley Ewer and *Clearing the Clutter* by Mary Lambert. However, if you're *really* keen to get started (good for you!) Mimi Tanner's popular e-book *Declutter Fast* is available for immediate download.

Your home is meant to be a place of refuge and relaxation. Don't make room for anything that robs you of more than it provides. Make a vow that 'selective' will be your new mindset. And before you know it, you will have busted your clutter and reclaimed your home.

## Set your own standards

If you are feeling seriously overwhelmed, it's vital that your schedule is based on *your standards*. If you're trying to attain levels of perfection to please other people, you may well lack the necessary motivation. But with responsibility comes power. So if the housework has been left in your hands, then *you* get to decide which jobs matter the most. Aim to prioritise what *you* feel is important.

If a 'significant other' takes issue with this, explain the situation, i.e., doing it your way will be an undoubted improvement on the status quo. Then give them your blessing to undertake any particular jobs they feel strongly about *themselves*. They may or may not decide that it's worth their effort, but either way, it's one less job for you to do.

For example, a friend of mine used to iron her partner's socks. She claimed he preferred them that way. However, when said partner was asked, if he lived alone, would he iron his own socks? - he said no. He admitted that he wasn't really *that* bothered. After that, his socks went un-ironed and he didn't have a (sockless) leg to stand on.

So, review your chores like a government troubleshooter. Trim the fat. Streamline. Have a policy of not doing for others anything that they wouldn't bother to do themselves (unless, of course, you actually *want* to...more on that later).

If you eliminate non-essential tasks, you will physically have less to do and mentally feel less overwhelmed. Thus you'll be much more able - and likely - to accomplish what you feel really does need doing.

# Reduce

Reducing your workload need not be about neglect or cutting corners. It can be about a more efficient use of limited resources, i.e., *you*.

There is only one you and there are only so many hours in the day. When you are overloaded with work - something's gotta give. The fact that you're reading this book suggests that this 'something' is currently your home or your mental health. Or both.

Time to prioritise, to determine which activities or objects you could happily do without - then ditch those instead.

## Simplify your life

Modern life can have us reeling in a frenzy of activity, often leaving us with the feeling that we're unable to cope. But how much of this urgency is really necessary? Yes, we are capable of extraordinary achievements - but not necessarily all at once and RIGHT NOW!

The website *The Slow Movement* uses the term 'time-poverty' to describe this uniquely modern issue. It suggests that, in our race to do, be, or have *something else*, we may be missing out on the simple pleasures of life. There are a number of cultural movements that address this problem and these are gaining momentum and popularity. (Leo Babauta's *Zen Habits* made *Time Magazine's* top ten blogs.) There is even a rise of new catch-phrases to communicate this phenomenon - downsizing, downshifting, decluttering. These all reflect a call to go back to basics, to slow down and simplify.

If your home has become a stress-infested work zone, perhaps it's time to reassess. Cast an enquiring eye over your home and your commitments. Consider all the areas that you devote your time/ life to - and make sure they're worth it. It is, literally, your life at stake.

> Let your boat of life be light, packed with only what you need - a homely home and simple pleasures.
>
> *Jerome K Jerome*

Simplifying your life and environment can be doubly effective in reducing overwhelm - giving you more time, and less to do. So, evaluate your life and simplify where you can. There is a calmer, happier you in there somewhere - by building some breathing space into your schedule, you are much more likely to find her.

## Retrain and conquer

Successful household management, like any other managerial task, requires training. Women are often expected to just 'know' this stuff. But as women's roles have evolved beyond the home, and families are increasingly far flung, we are missing out on much of the wisdom that used to be passed down from female relations.

There are generations of women - the daughters of feminism - who grew up being told they had so much more to offer than domestic servitude. As a result they shunned (if it was offered) the education that women had previously received in the home, i.e., *how to run a home.* I'll admit that, as a girl, I'd have met any 'handy hints' with scorn and derision. *I don't need to know that stuff - I'm going places!* Yet even career women have homes to keep. The difference is that now we have to do it without adequate training.

No wonder we're feeling overwhelmed - so much to do and we haven't a clue!

But this essential knowledge still exists. The training we need *is* still available - and it's information that could really help us. We may now have to go 'out there' and find it - but this is a step worth taking. Acquiring this knowledge could make our homes and lives run much more smoothly.

So, make it your mission to seek out expert advice, trade secrets, and efficient techniques. Research any proven time-savers or lessons passed down over generations. Buy or borrow books, learn from the professionals - benefit from others' experience. Surf the web - a lot of great information is available free of charge. You may even find yourself inspired and motivated, as well as educated. (I find I'm always spurred into action after a quick flick through *The Cleaning Bible* by those Queens of Clean, Kim and Aggie.)

There are many tricks and tips that could radically reduce your workload and it's definitely worth the initial time investment to explore and implement them. Getting clued up on these shortcuts could knock hours off your weekly routine - which over the course of a lifetime could translate to *years*!

So why not research, learn and adopt these time-tested labour-saving techniques? We will spend a significant portion of our lives doing unavoidable housework - let's cut out any unnecessary stuff.

# Delegate

The first rule of management is delegation.
Don't try and do everything yourself
because you can't.

*Anthea Turner, author of* The Perfect Housewife

There are three reasons to delegate:

★ You can't physically do all that needs to be done.

★ You don't want to do certain tasks.

★ Your talents are better utilised elsewhere.

One, two or even all of these conditions may apply to your housework schedule. Yet delegation is something many women struggle with. Call us control freaks, but we tend to believe that only we can do it the right way - Our Way. This may be true, but if you are frazzled and overwhelmed, then *good enough* is good enough.

Although we may be notoriously wonderful at multi-tasking, we haven't yet learned how to clone ourselves, and there is only so much a single person can do. So if you're struggling with more than you can cope with, it's time to call for reinforcements. No one will think any less of you if you accept a little help. In fact, many of the world's greatest achievers have become great partly because of their ability to delegate.

But within the home, which jobs should you delegate? And to whom?

Well, firstly, the most effective tactic in delegation, indeed for success in all walks of life, is - do what you do best. Stick to your strengths. This is not only a more healthful and satisfying strategy - it's more efficient. When you excel at a certain task you are naturally more motivated and productive. When you enjoy your work, you make a better job of it.

So, consider your chores, and pick your favourites. Select the jobs you don't mind, maybe even enjoy. (If you loathe them all, however, you're going to have to find the ways and means for some major delegation - but this could still be the right thing for you.)

We all have varying strengths, talents and preferences, and it makes sense for us to work with, rather than against, them. So, in our plan to conquer overwhelm - with the aim of reducing your workload - you might as well delegate the bits that you like the least.

Everyone has a job that they mysteriously never get round to. Mine is mopping. Whenever it occurs to me that the floor really does need cleaning, I suddenly find something else very urgent to do. If you live alone, you can leave it as long as you can bear it. If you don't, you may as well admit your terminal procrastination and take steps to delegate.

When you have a schedule that you can physically manage and that doesn't make you want to run screaming from the house, you'll be far more likely to cope productively. Plus you'll be infinitely happier (a bonus not to be underestimated). But you're probably wondering, *What about the other stuff? Who will do all the jobs that I find boring, loathsome or intolerable?*

Believe it or not - some people enjoy doing the things you can't or don't want to do. One person's work may be another person's play. There are people who actually love to cook and clean and are great at it! (No really, it's true!)

So if you're prepared to relinquish a little control (and hard work) and delegate the jobs you don't like, the next question becomes - who to delegate to?

## To hire or not to hire...?

When it comes to hiring domestic help, there are women who do (or would) and women who don't, and won't.

If any of the latter group are suffering from overwhelm, it may be time to reconsider. As for the rest of us, again we fall into two camps, those who hire (in which case, I salute you but you can skip this section) and those who can't find the resources or justify the expense. So let's just explore that a little...

In his book, *The Success Principles*, Jack Canfield writes, 'Most female executives spend too much time running their household, when they could easily and inexpensively delegate this task to a cleaning service or part-time mother's helper, freeing themselves to focus on their career or spend more time with their family.'

This is sound advice for female executives, but may also apply to any working women. If you're in paid employment, it's a simple matter of economics. Put a value on your time - if it's more than you would pay for staff (and you don't loathe your job even more than the housework), it makes sense to work those extra hours at your job and pay someone else to clean your home. You can't do both simultaneously, so do the one you prefer.

There's a slightly different argument for the Stay-At-Homes. My husband once (and only once) suggested, that since I was at home all day - surely I could do all the housework? He was reluctant to pay for work when I was 'available' to do it. I claimed that I'd given up my career to raise children, not dust ornaments, but my reluctance wasn't an availability issue, more a motivational problem. For the sake of marital harmony, though, we chose to agree to disagree. (He's good like that.)

However, I have since found that, in this scenario, the most effective argument for domestic help is the case study of a good friend.

Beth was a full-time mum to two children under three. She herself had very high standards for her home but was increasingly feeling the strain of all the housework, on top of the childcare. Her husband refused to entertain the idea of a cleaner. He claimed it was an unnecessary expense that they couldn't afford. Beth soldiered on, becoming more and more frazzled and stressed out. Her health began to suffer. This went on for quite a while, but ultimately, something had to give. Struggling to maintain her own exacting standards - without assistance - Beth ended up in hospital following a collapse.

There she had a kind of epiphany: *she needed help*. Given the circumstances, her husband was inclined to agree. (During her spell in hospital, her husband had to shell out far more cash in emergency childcare than it would have cost him to hire a cleaner for years!) These days,

> Asking for help is not a sign of weakness but a sign of strength.
>
> *Proverb*

Beth delegates without guilt and is healthier and happier. The family finances soon adjusted to the *necessary* expense. Now her home is kept to her satisfaction, yet she's not killing herself to achieve it.

There's a saying that people who don't have time for exercise will be forced to find time for illness. Similarly, if you don't find the resources for some badly needed relief, ultimately you're going to burn out.

So don't wait until you're at the point of collapse (or divorce) to justify some help. After all, prevention is better than cure. Hiring some support is not a luxury or extravagance if your sanity, well-being or relationships are on the line. When it comes to the quality of your life, getting some help may be a lifesaver you can't afford to do without.

Whatever path you have chosen - family, career, or both - you deserve a work/life ratio that doesn't leave you on the brink of exhaustion. (I know from experience that a home does not look its best when the Lady of the House is in hospital.) In the workplace, work/life-balance is the new buzzword for success. All those high-powered execs heading for burnout are opting to downsize. But, if finances allow, why should women who devote their lives to their families not be entitled to the same basic need - that of balance?

> Now, as always, the most automated appliance in a household is the mother.
>
> *Beverly Jones*

Hiring help, then, can be a sound investment in your mental and physical health. But it can also be money well spent in terms of family harmony. There is an emotional and psychological element to cleaning up other people's mess. If you are always the cleaner and they are always the 'messers', this can really affect your relationships. It's easy to see how resentments can occur, even with those you love. (Watching someone carelessly wee all over a toilet you've just cleaned is *really annoying* – even if that someone is only 2½.)

So, opting for help is not a purely selfish endeavour. The entire household will undoubtedly benefit, if only from the reduced friction.

NOTE: If hiring help would involve financial stress or difficulty or incur more problems than it would alleviate, then maybe now is not the time. But if you decide you have the will, I believe you can find a way. In the meantime, fear not! Read on to discover some cost-free alternatives a little closer to home...

## Keep it in the family

If, for whatever reason, you don't take on external help (and even if you do - you'll still have to tidy up before they come!), it makes sense to utilise existing labour sources. I'm referring to the Others. The people you live with. Now you may be thinking - if those we live with did their fair share, we wouldn't need this book! But I believe it's possible (and just) to recruit them in your domestic battle. It's simply a case of finding the right approach...

Time to reconsider your family members, and to view them as potential allies, rather than the enemy. (The following techniques are aimed at those with partners and/or children. However these principles are based on human nature and so could be applied to any form of [human] housemate.)

The following ideas are ways to encourage/coerce/bribe/trick family members into helping out, but this is not an immoral scheme. Neither is it taking an unfair advantage. You're just redressing an imbalance. Those you live with a) undoubtedly add to your workload, and b) (hopefully) care about your well-being. So you shouldn't feel any guilt in enlisting their assistance (whether they are aware of it or not).

Besides, you can't force people to do anything they don't want to, for long. The trick is to get them to *want* to do it. So, here are a few simple tactics to make your housemates more willing (and more likely) to help out in the home.

**Make a start**. If you *just begin*, strange things happen. People see what you're doing and, bizarrely, they often want to be in on it. For example, if I make a start on the carnage that is my sons' bedroom (making sure they're present), they magically say, 'Can we help you, Mummy?'

Similarly, if my husband is hanging round the kitchen and I run a sink full of hot soapy water, before *mysteriously* disappearing... when I return, he's got his hands in the sink! This one baffles me but I'm happy to go with it. Give it a go - at the very worst you've got the job started (which can often be the hardest part).

**Be visible.** Your efforts in the home will be valued, not by what you *actually* do, but by what the Others *notice* that you do. A favourite trick of mine is to beaver away with all the chores whilst family members are around to see it. Then I take my Me-Time when they're all out. (I'm pretty sure they forget I even exist when they're off 'doing their thing', so they're not likely to wonder what I've been up to.)

If your family's awareness of you consists of the busy person, caring for them and looking after the home, your efforts will be logged, both consciously and subconsciously. And when they feel that you do plenty for them, they will be naturally more inclined to help - they may even volunteer. (Hope springs eternal...)

**Don't nag.** I wish I had learned this years ago: nagging is counter-productive. I'll say that again - nagging is *counter*-productive. Not only will it not yield the assistance you're after, but it has the opposite effect! It creates resentment, making people *less* likely to want to help you.

Most people actually get enjoyment from helping others, but *only* if they believe it was their idea. *Not* if they were bullied into it. You want your family to enjoy helping, if only because then they'll be far more likely to pitch in again in future. So try a lighter-hearted approach, and prepare to be amazed.

**Ask.** People are not psychic. You may assume that they know, or ought to know, what you require of them. In reality, though, they often don't. So, tell them! If you outline your expectations, coming to an agreement in a calm and pleasant manner *before it becomes an issue*, they are much more likely to oblige than if they are harangued by a frazzled banshee. (Plus they also have less excuse for not doing their bit...)

**Appreciate.** Two very small words can go a long, long way: *Thank you*. Every single person on the planet wants to be appreciated. It really counts for a lot. And it is so easy to do! Though you may already appreciate it when someone helps out, if you don't *let them know*, you are missing a powerful opportunity to a) increase your bond with that person, and b) encourage them to help you the next time.

Perhaps you feel that they ought to do it without thanks, and you may be right. But how much more inclined would you feel to do your duties, if you knew they were appreciated?

**Play swaps.** Just maybe, the jobs you hate are fun to somebody else. And vice versa. For example, my nine-year-old son finds ironing very exciting. (He's a boy, there's a gadget involved...) I am less inclined toward the mountain of clean-but-crumpled clothes that need attention. On the other hand, he hates sorting out his toys, which appeals to my ordered brain. So we happily swap. It's a great arrangement that gets the work done and also instills a spirit of teamwork and cooperation. (Though I've yet to find someone to barter with for the toilet cleaning...)

**Just mention it.** I am constantly surprised by the power of simply mentioning a need or a wish - and this applies to life, not just housework. Just by commenting on my requirements, it's amazing how things 'coincidentally' work out in my favour. For example, I may casually remark that I really love it when the bedroom floor is free of dirty clothes. Then later, as my husband is about to scatter his clothes where he may, he mysteriously pauses, then veers towards the laundry basket!

I know it sounds dubious but there's a complex Jungian theory for this phenomenon (called 'synchronicity') which makes for fascinating, though mind-boggling, study (if you like that sort of thing). However, I don't need to understand it to use it and enjoy the benefits. Try it, it's fun!

**Offer rewards**. When all else fails, get down to what everybody understands - bribery. This is a particularly effective tactic with young children, who can't see benefits beyond their immediate needs. Sometimes you have to offer/withhold something they really want in order to get them to do something you really want.

The extent to which you employ this measure is a matter for you and your conscience...

## A word about child labour

The job of a parent involves raising children to be valuable members of society - people who can not only look after themselves, but also have an empathy for the needs of others. It is only right and fair that they learn to contribute. So banish any guilt you may have about putting your children to work!

(Obviously, this principle assumes responsible judgement and that you have no desire to exploit your children and give them unsuitable tasks, such as sending them up chimneys, etc...)

This practice not only helps to alleviate some of your workload, but you're actually doing your children, and their future families, a favour. And start young! Children are more likely to embrace the concepts of independence and helpfulness if they become a habit from an early age. For example, if you have a policy that your children *earn* their pocket money (with age-appropriate tasks) - you will instill a work ethic that will stand them in good stead for the rest of their lives. And children *love* responsibility! It boosts their confidence and self-esteem, and gives them a sense of achievement and pride.

Besides, what may seem like a tedious chore to you may have a novelty factor for a child. Children see everything as an opportunity to play. They're not in a rush or preoccupied. They've got time to find the fun. In my house, give a child a cloth and a (non-toxic) spray bottle, point them in the direction of your grubbiest surfaces, and it's smiles all round!

23

It's a great idea to buy younger children miniature cooking and cleaning equipment, so they can copy you as you cook or clean. Children love to mimic and it's how they learn. (I struggle to vacuum without one of my boys following me round with a toy version.) You'll be simultaneously entertaining and bonding with your offspring whilst training future assistants. This practice will also provide your children with a valuable sense of the time and effort required in taking care of a home.

> Never help a child with a task at which he feels he can succeed.
>
> *Maria Montessori*

Please be aware, however, that if you decide to encourage your children to help around the house, it is necessary to take the long view. You may often feel that it'd be easier to do a job yourself, and on each single occasion, it most likely would be. But if you persevere, eventually, they'll know what to do and will be able to do it by themselves. This will reap dividends in the long run. The help and assistance they provide in future years will make the training period worthwhile.

*N.B.* Children, like adults, respond better to jobs which have visible or measurable results. Reward charts are particularly effective with younger children. (It's amazing what a child will do for a sticker!)

## Delegate to the inanimate

It's not only our fellow humans who can prevent us drowning in domesticity. Technological advances have changed the lot of homemakers immeasurably. For example, few of us now have to devote *a whole day* to washing. But we can, and should, take more advantage of these developments wherever possible.

Here you can exploit with abandon! There are no relationships to consider or feelings to be spared (although I swear my dishwasher performs better when I talk nicely to it...).

**If you've got it - use it!** I have a friend who only uses her dishwasher at Christmas. Her husband insists it's a waste of water and that it's actually easier to wash the dishes, than to load, unload, and so on. (Arguably, either way is easy for him, as he leaves it all to his wife...) As I have said before, with responsibility comes power. If you're doing the job - you get to do it *your way*. So, if you'd like to enlist electronic assistance, then do.

Equally, if you prefer to wash by hand, again, it's your decision.

However, please don't give yourself extra work out of misplaced ideas of wastefulness. Washing dishes by hand uses approximately three times the water used by a dishwasher cycle. Appliances are usually more efficient than the equivalent human effort - that's why they were invented! So, in making use of your dishwasher, you'll be saving your time *and* the planet (not to mention your hands).

**Keep up to date.** Be alert to new time-saving devices or energy-efficient inventions. My current favourite is the Robot Vacuum Cleaner. (There are both reasonable and blow-the-budget versions.) This little poppet pootles around your home, sucking up all the debris until the poor thing is exhausted - at which point he (I like to think of it as male) takes himself back to his little charging station. It's probably not the greatest technological advance but think of the man/woman-hours to be saved across the world! In fact, one reviewer was so enamoured with this device, he was uncertain who he'd save first in the event of a fire - his wife or his RoboVac? (I bet Mrs Reviewer was chuffed to bits with this dubious gesture...)

There is also a sister product newly available, the Scooba robotic mop. It's been getting some rave reviews but I have yet to enjoy its services. (Santa, if you're listening...)

So haul your housework into the digital age. Keep an eye out for anything that could help automate your workload. There are TV shows and magazines devoted to the latest tech inventions, whilst websites are great for honest reviews that cut through the marketing hype.

**Mouse power.** Internet shopping. Whether or not you're a dedicated surfer, there are benefits to using this technology. Possibly the most time- (and back-) saving of these is getting your regular groceries delivered. Now you may actually enjoy the supermarket experience, the casual browsing, meandering up and down the aisles, etc... If so, you can still opt to venture out *as the mood takes you.* But for those boring, essential (and bulky or heavy) items - why not get them delivered? I, for one, find no joy in lugging loo rolls and washing detergent to and from my car.

So set up a list of those recurring weekly or monthly items and have someone else haul them from store to door. And if anyone tells you that's lazy, tell them it's not. It's efficient outsourcing. So there.

# What mess?

I have been a student of *feng shui* for a number of years. Though some of the principles can be quite complex, one notion that I came across struck me with its wonderful simplicity (not to mention its potential for application to a messy home).

The particular nugget of enlightenment was this: The negative effects of elements that create Poison Arrows, Missing Corners, or Inauspicious Chi, etc, are all diminished... if you can't see them.

So even if you have some evil chi gathering in pockets in your home, you can rob it of its power (over you) by simply *not seeing it*.

Can you spot the potential for (temporary) relief? For example, if you're too utterly exhausted to tackle the playroom - just close the door! Or if your spare room is a little frightening - don't go in there! You literally make things worse by looking at it - so don't!

Out of sight, out of mind.

*Proverb*

Obviously the applications are limited, i.e., you can't stay out of the kitchen forever. Also, the mess will undoubtedly still be there when you do next venture in (though miracles do happen...). But until you can deal with it, don't torture yourself with the sight of it.

This simple practice will reduce your feelings of overwhelm and plug a leak of your precious mental energy, which you can then devote to more pressing matters.

# Bite the bullet

If you're fighting a losing battle that you simply cannot win, stop fighting!

There comes a point when it makes sense to deploy more rational (and healthier) tactics such as acceptance, patience and tolerance. These may not always be the easiest option (sometimes, bizarrely, we *prefer* to get upset), but it can be done. And it can be as simple as making the decision to do so.

You can actually *decide* to refuse to let something bug you. Even the phrase *'let* it bug you' implies that we have the power to choose - which we do!

In deciding to not rise to the bait, you regain control. Perhaps you can't control the state of the house/family/life, etc, - but you *can* control how it affects you. You are in control of how you react. A person or circumstance can only annoy you with your permission. And where does 'being annoyed' get you anyway?

Richard Carlson (author of *Don't Sweat the Small Stuff (and It's All Small Stuff)* offers this advice: 'Gently remind yourself that life is okay the way it is, right now. In the absence of your judgement, everything would be fine.'

If you decide to practice more acceptance of the things you can't control - they may still happen, but they will bother you less. Then you can devote your energy to the areas where you *can* make a difference.

So, learn to recognise those instances when you cannot win. Accept those inalienable truths: Children will leave out their toys. People will make crumbs in your kitchen. There will always be laundry.

Stop fighting the inevitable. Embrace acceptance. This is not defeat. This is enlightened housekeeping.

God grant me
the serenity to
accept the things
I cannot change,
the courage
to change
the things I can,
and the wisdom
to know
the difference.

*Serenity Prayer*

# Let battle commence!

Once you have eliminated, reduced, delegated, ignored or accepted
what you can - it's time to cope with what's left...

# Baby Steps

It is better to take many small steps
in the right direction
than to make a great leap forward
only to stumble back.

*Chinese proverb*

One piece of advice that changed my whole approach to housework was from the wonderful 'FlyLady' website. Among many other useful insights, FlyLady highlights the delusional nature of those of us who say things like, *I won't pick up that item yet, as I'll do a proper tidy-up later.* Or, *I'll leave that spill for now because I'm going to have a* Big Kitchen Clean *tomorrow.* Of course, those mammoth sessions are few and far between and in the meantime, the work is heading dangerously towards overwhelming levels.

So the sage FlyLady's advice is to take baby steps. Avoid the 'all or nothing' mindset. In other words (and borrowing from a certain sporting goods manufacturer): Just do it! Just do that one little job. After all, overwhelm only arises from the *accumulation* of little jobs which have been left un-done.

## Little and Often

This 'Little and Often' technique is a favourite among professional housekeepers - because it works! Plus, it's much easier to motivate yourself to do a small job than to find the strength for a Herculean effort. And it can be more efficient - because you deal with jobs as they arise (many jobs become more time-consuming the longer they are left). But perhaps most importantly in cases of overwhelm, any action, however small, will help you feel that you're still in control.

There is another hidden power to this strategy, which lies in what it prevents - the chance to think *too much* about your housework.

For example, I have a friend who spends one day a week cleaning her whole house. One full day! Her son is at nursery two days a week, so one of her precious pockets of peace is spent doing housework. This obviously works for her, and each to their own. But for women of a certain mindset it's a recipe for resentment and frustration.

I am one such woman. If I were to spend a whole day cleaning, that small voice in my head would be grumbling, *What a waste of a day. I really don't want to be doing this. I hate spending so much time on housework. I'd much rather be doing x,y and z....* Even after the work was done, I'd still begrudge the time spent, because within hours, the house would no longer be spotless. So where were the fruits of a whole day's labour?

A journey of 1000 miles must begin with a single step.

*Lao-Tzu*

If you are subject to similar depressing and destructive musings, the baby steps approach will help to nip them in the bud. These mini-efforts may (or may not) amount to more than one full day's labour, but it's the psychological impact that we're concerned with here. Your mental state dictates the state of your home, health and sanity. More important than cutting your housework time, is ensuring you emerge with your mental health intact.

However, if you love to immerse yourself in a Great Big Clean and that works for you, by all means, stick with it. But be aware that spending large chunks of time on domestic work opens up *a lot* of potential for the negative brain-chatter to kick in. And be honest - if you're so overwhelmed with chores, will you really find the necessary time, energy or inclination?

## The '3-Sees' Rule

Let's imagine you notice a little something that needs doing. But you don't do it. Maybe you have a valid reason - you're rushing out, you have a child in your arms, the phone's ringing, dinner's burning, etc. That's okay, that's real life. So you leave it, for now. However, you will have mentally logged it, so the next time you see it, instead of thinking, *Oh, that needs doing,* this time you think, *Oh, no, not that again.*

That small task has turned into a minor annoyance. So do you do it the second time? Again you may have good reasons to not do it yet or, if you're like me, you may be tempted to just leave it. But there is a saying that what you resist, persists. In other words - that little job isn't going anywhere.

By the third time you see it, it will be costing you emotional and mental energy, out of all proportion to the actual task. So you pay a price for dodging those little jobs. *Not* doing them costs you thought-units - they sap your mental energy. And if you have a number of little tasks that need attention, you are heading for overwhelm. Every time you see each one, your heart sinks a little. If they build up, your heart can sink to depths from which it can be hard to recover.

So the next time you notice a small task, ask yourself - do I have a good reason to not do it *right now?* If you do - you can neglect it without guilt or self-recrimination. (Besides, you'll most likely get a second chance...) But if you don't have a good reason, either the first or second time - take care of it! Then it will never bother you again! You will be saved the stress of seeing it over and over. This is how you will win the war against overwhelm - one small battle at a time.

If this sounds like hard work (and you are keen to avoid hard work), it can be motivating to remember that if you leave it, *it will probably take you longer, later.*

Think of clutter, stains, food spills, etc. It might take 5 seconds to remove a dried-on, soaked-in spill from a surface, where it would have only taken 1 second had it been done immediately. Okay, it's only a difference of 4 seconds but actually, the job has increased in time required by 400%! Haven't you got enough to do, without increasing your labour-time? If you're swamped with work, time-efficiency is your friend. So, if possible, do jobs when they can be done quickest - which is usually sooner rather than later.

> Procrastination is the art of keeping up with yesterday.
>
> *Don Marquis*

There are even jobs that can reach a point of no return. For example, if you leave the vacuuming long enough, the dust and dirt will actually be ground into the carpet fibres and destroy them. Your carpet will, literally, never be the same again.

So make it a rule that you will deal with the little jobs as you notice them. Maybe not the first time (if you have a *good* reason), but hopefully the second time or absolutely, positively, no excuses, by the third time you see it. Make a solemn pledge, this moment - there is power in commitment. Vow to shoot down the little joblings as they come up.

It's in your own best interests, I promise.

## The power of a minute

Sixty seconds. It doesn't seem like a lot. For the mountain of work before you, one minute wouldn't even make a dent, right? Wrong. Let's say you had an hour, a day, a week? Could you get all the work done then? Let's hope so! But what are those time frames made of? Minutes. What is life made of? Minutes!

Today's media is rife with strategies that harness the power of the single minute. You can even take a one-minute vacation! And according to Robert Allen and Mark Victor Hansen in their hugely successful book, *The One Minute Millionaire*, 'You can become a millionaire, one minute at a time.' Surely getting on top of your chores is easier than making a million dollars? (Though just think of the domestic assistance you could buy...)

So if the thought of spending a day, an afternoon, or an hour wreaks havoc with your brain, use a little Minute Magic. To get you started, here are a few suggestions of jobs that can usually be done in a minute.

* ★ Empty the kitchen bin
* ★ Give the toilet a wipe-over
* ★ Plan the dinner
* ★ Write a grocery list
* ★ Sort a pile of papers
* ★ Put in a laundry load
* ★ Run a sink of hot soapy water
* ★ Unload the dishwasher
* ★ Polish a mirror
* ★ Dust the TV
* ★ Clear the kitchen table

So, the next time you look at a job and think, *Oh, I haven't got time to do it now*, give yourself a challenge. Ask, *Could it be done in a minute?* If the answer is yes, and you have a minute to spare - get it done! A minute later, you'll have one less irritating chore to bug you. This is the minute-by-minute route out of overwhelm.

When you face jobs head on, they tend to take far less time than you imagine. And doing those minor jobs instead of procrastinating about them will relieve so much mental energy. You will feel more capable and effective and possibly lighter! So that annoying chore that you dispatch in the work of moments could be the most satisfying minute you spend all day.

# Getting started

Often this where we come unstuck.

If getting started is hard for you, take comfort in the fact that you are not alone. Some of the greatest minds in history have recognised the difficulty in just getting going. Pythagoras went as far as to say, 'The beginning is half the whole.'

However, if you're overwhelmed by the sheer volume of chores, it may not be starting a job that's the problem, but knowing which job to start! So here are a few ideas on how to select which ones to do first (i.e., at all). Once you've covered the fundamental hygiene bases and no one's health is at stake, it's really a matter of personal preference. There are many varied systems and theories on efficiency and productivity, but on home territory you get to choose. So simply pick the strategy that works for you...

**Do your favourite job first.** We're more likely to do the jobs we enjoy than ever get round to that loathsome, hated task which we feel very strongly about avoiding. So, why fight it? Go with it. Do your favourites first. That way, you're guaranteed to at least get something done. If the first job on your list makes you want to go back to bed, it doesn't bode well for the rest of the day.

**Do your least favourite job first.** This theory is the exact opposite of the above, but it seems to work for some people. In Brian Tracy's book about procrastination, *Eat That Frog*, he suggests doing your most hated task first. His reasoning is that in doing so, the rest of the day can only improve.

Though I can see the logic in this, it's not for me. If my first job of the day was to mop the floor, there's a real danger I might give up after breakfast and go shopping – probably not the most productive approach. But if this appeals to your sense of getting the worst over with, line up your frogs and tuck in!

**Do the most satisfying job first** Sometimes, you may not like the task but you absolutely love the result. (For me this applies to the majority of the housework schedule...) So, pick a job that will give you the most satisfaction *when it is done*. For example, you may not be over-enamoured with cleaning the toilet. However, it becomes more tolerable when you factor in that happy sense of satisfaction when a visitor asks to use your loo - and you know it's spotless.

# Keep a sense of perspective

John Lennon famously wondered, *Why on earth are we here? Surely,* he ventured, *not to live in pain and fear?*

I would add: surely not to spend our life either doing housework or stressing over it? Feeling overwhelmed is not our natural state - something has gone wrong. It's possible that what's needed to fix it is a fresh perspective.

So, when you're overwhelmed with housework, it can be helpful to remember that there is more to life...

**The Great Outdoors.** Go outside. Get back to nature. See things bigger than your own life. If you're getting bogged down with the minutiae of everyday life, it's time to step back and see the bigger picture. To get a true sense of what's important, look at the vastness of the sea or sky or mountains.

How much does the state of one home really matter in the grand scheme of things?

**The Young Ones.** Spend time with children - they know instinctively what's important. They may not know (or care!) the price of anything but they know the *value* of everything. They worry less about what they should do and concentrate on what makes them happy. It's a refreshing way to live and one that could benefit you if life has lost its sparkle. Children may have much to learn, but they also have much to teach.

So, take a tip from the young ones - do things just for fun. Remember how to play. It's not wasting time - it's living!

**The Not-So-Young Ones.** Chat with someone older and wiser. Many of the world's most civilised cultures revere the elderly because of the many lessons they've learned through the experience of their lifetimes. So why not benefit from their lessons and experience?

Don't wait till the end of your own lifetime to look back and realise what was important. Find out now. Or you just might miss it.

# Section 2:

# Injustice

# It's just not fair!

A sense of justice is part of human nature. It's inherent in our make-up to want things to be fair. So when an injustice occurs, it can really get under our skin, often out of all proportion to the original offence. Perhaps there are occasions in your domestic life when it's not the chores, as such, that drive you mad - it's the infuriating injustice of *it always being down to you.*

So, unfairness instinctively bothers us and we are programmed to try and rectify it. But by a cruel twist of whatever force is in charge, fairness is not always the natural order of things. Often, quite simply, life isn't fair.

> Expecting the world to treat you fairly because you're a good person is a little like expecting a bull not to attack you because you're a vegetarian.
>
> Dennis Wholey

As a child, I remember hearing the 'life's not fair' line, whenever I bemoaned some injustice or other to my parents. This 'explanation' would be issued as an end to the discussion. Back then, it was rare that I'd accept this as reasonable or concede defeat. (I was what you might call a willful child...) In recent years, however, I have come to (begrudgingly) accept that my parents were right - life comes with no promise of fairness.

Which leaves us with the question: How do we marry our justice-seeking instincts with an unjust world?

## Be solution-focused

One powerful remedy to feelings of injustice is to become solution-focused. According to recent scientific discoveries, when you give your attention to something, you are actually programming your brain to notice more instances of it.

So, by dwelling on a certain domestic injustice, going over and over it, you are training yourself to be super-sensitive to that problem. You are hard-wiring your brain to be on the lookout for similar treatment. Unfortunately this means that, the more you focus on being unfairly treated, the more you'll become aware of that treatment in all areas of your life.

You may even have seen evidence of this. Do you know anyone who feels that the world is against them? They are victimised by almost everyone they meet. And the more they bemoan all their injustices - the more they get to moan about!

Ironically, this just isn't fair! But it's a result of the filters in our brain called the RAS – the Reticular Activating System. It's a fascinating phenomenon and once you know about it, you can use it to help you - rather than obliviously allowing it to hold you back. (There's more on this coming up, but for more extensive information on RAS theory, *Having It All* by John Assaraf contains a great introduction to the subject.)

Successful people know this principle, i.e., what you focus on, you get more of. Although some may not know or recognise it consciously, it is undoubtedly a contributor to their success. Instead of staying stuck in the rut of a problem, successful people develop a solution-oriented approach. They don't dwell on what's gone wrong. Instead, they turn all their attention and energy to what needs to be done to make it right. They harness the power of their brain filters and solutions start popping up all over the place.

So if you'd like to successfully reduce your feelings of being unfairly treated, follow their example. By all means, *identify* the problem, that's an essential step in solving it. But once you've done that - *start focusing on the solution.*

## Fight, flight...or accept?

In seeking a solution to any injustice, you have three options: try to change the situation, leave the situation, or accept the situation. You may disagree with me here, claiming that you are trapped by your circumstances, but there is always something you can do, even if it's just to change your reaction or approach. Whilst you may be unable to control other people's behaviour, you can control how much you allow it to effect you. Even if you simply reach a new acceptance or tolerance, that in itself is a change.

You may also balk at the idea of accepting unjust treatment and I'll admit, these have been some difficult lessons for me. But could it be possible that your perception of an injustice is only one way of looking at it? In some cases, where we're suffering a perceived injustice, it may be that a different viewpoint will bring a new, less-aggrieved perspective. It's possible that considering your particular bugbear from a different angle will make it a little easier to tolerate.

So, rather than struggling against outer circumstances beyond your control, an attitude shift may be the answer. Open yourself up to those *I never thought of it like that* moments. You'll be amazed by the relief and mental calm that arises when you let go of the need to feel mistreated. And the benefits of making peace with your domestic gripes can have far-reaching effects across every aspect of your life.

*You can never solve a problem on the level on which it was created.*

*Albert Einstein*

Of course, there may be occasions when you aren't imagining it - it really isn't fair! But again, that's life. For those times, you'll have to choose for yourself whether to change, accept, or leave the situation. I believe the ideal scenario will be to find a balance between what should rightly be kicked against and what could be if not accepted, then at least tolerated.

Convinced? I didn't think so. But read on with an open mind and prepare to be a little less angry with your lot.

Q: Why should I?

A: Maybe you shouldn't, but…

# Letting go

So, life isn't always fair. Deep down, you know that. But do you accept it? Or do you struggle on with battles that you can never win?

Of course, there may be occasions that you feel so strongly, you simply cannot or will not admit defeat - however futile the battle. If it would eat you up to *not* react - then that may be your particular crusade, your vital issue, where acceptance is not an option.

That alone is not such a bad thing - the world is a better place for the good people who have railed against injustice. It's certainly true that some battles are worth fighting.

The trouble comes when we start to fight every battle going, no matter how minor or inconsequential. This can lead to much friction and disharmony, not to mention emotional exhaustion. Though you may be claiming victories for your principles - at what price?

So how do you know which battles to fight and which to accept? Well, the good news is - you get to choose! In fact, you probably already know, instinctively, which battles you simply have to fight. However, if you want to have the energy (and impact) for the battles that really matter, you'll need to relinquish some of your minor griefs.

In the words of Sun Tzu, author of the insightful classic, *The Art of War*: 'Choose your battles wisely. Do not fight battles you cannot win.'

> Pick battles
> big enough
> to matter,
> small enough
> to win.
>
> *Jonathan Kozol*

Letting go of a few petty grievances is not weakness or defeat - it is empowering. *You* are the one who will benefit the most. In fact, you may be surprised by how liberating this can be.

We humans tend to hold on to far too many grudges and this only does us harm. Or, as the Buddha eloquently put it: 'Holding on to anger is like grasping a hot coal with the intent of throwing it at someone else; you are the one who gets burned.' So, releasing unnecessary negative mental energy will have positive implications for *your* health and happiness.

It makes sense, then, to choose your battles wisely and, for your own sake, let go of the ones that don't really matter. It can help to remember this, in the heat of your next injustice. First of all, question whether it's actually a battle you can win. But even then, ask yourself, *Is this really a battle worth taking on? Do I want to fight this, even though it could damage my relationships or my health? Could I let this one go?* The simple act of pausing before you react will, in itself, defuse some of your anger which will, by default, benefit *you* greatly.

However, there may be times when you ask, *Could I let this go?* - and the answer is *No!* Despite the logical arguments for rising above the unimportant battles, in practice, it's not always easy. Your head may decide to surrender a losing battle, or that it's not that big a deal, but there may be times when the heart doesn't oblige. Or you may still be irritated by minor griefs which you decided to leave un-fought. Be prepared for this; you're only human.

One consolation is that acceptance and forgiveness become easier with practice. They are skills which can be learned and refined. What feels impossibly difficult at first will one day be automatic (and your life will be greatly improved as a result).

> Just remember,
> when you should
> grab something,
> grab it;
> when you should
> let go, let go.
>
> *Anon.*

There are also a number of specialist methods which you can learn, called releasing techniques. An increasingly popular and effective process is *Emotional Freedom Techniques* (EFT) which works on your body's energy channels to alleviate negative emotions. Another technique is the *Sedona Method*, which is a process of asking yourself a few simple questions. (Don't be fooled by the simplicity of this. It's a highly effective programme which has changed many lives for the better.)

These are just a couple of my favourite techniques, but there are many others. If you feel you'd benefit from external help, do a little research and look into whichever method appeals the most to you. There is a wealth of support available, primarily because these skills don't come naturally to most people! But don't let the fact that it doesn't come naturally trick you into believing it won't benefit you. (We are masters at self-sabotage.)

Despite the initial effort, developing an ability to 'let it go' may just be the best thing you ever do - for yourself.

# Being right vs being happy

Okay, so it may not be fair. It may not be down to you to pick up the socks that couldn't make it to the laundry basket. You may have done the dishes six times this week and surely somebody else could make an effort, etc... etc... But, in the words of some rapper or other - What you gonna do?

Well, in the face of all this 'mistreatment', there is one element that you can control - *your reaction*. A situation may be unfair, but it is possible to come to terms with it, to rise above the injustice, in the pursuit of a higher goal. You can decide which is more important to you: justice or peace?

## Where does anger get you?

It may be true that you *shouldn't have to* pick up the Others' clothes from the floor but let's just ignore that fact for a moment. (This is surprisingly easy to do: just *choose* to not get mad. It can sometimes be simple as that!) If you pick up the offending item and drop it in the laundry bin, without the usual ranting and grumbling, it will cost *you* so much less in mental energy and negative emotions. You may be justified in getting angry - but anger is bad for *you*. So you are allowing that minor annoyance to take an even greater toll on your well-being. Now that really is unfair.

> The severest justice may not always be the best policy.
>
> Abraham Lincoln

To illustrate my claim, I offer you a true-life example, courtesy of my domestic situation. My husband has an unusual technique when it comes to reading the newspaper in the bath. You may think, there is only one way to read a newspaper (front to back), or possibly two (sports pages first). But, as far as I am aware, my beloved is the only person on the planet who reads the newspaper - leaf by leaf!

Allow me to demonstrate, in a 32-page paper, he will first read page 1, then page 2. So far, so conventional. However, he will then separate those pages from the main body, to read pages 31 and 32. I know, absolutely bonkers. Even his mother admits to a disappointed bafflement. It is, in fact, such an illogical procedure that he often reads the latter section of a story before the first bit! Now, you may just dismiss this as eccentricity, or an endearing idiosyncrasy, were it not for the fact that after his bath, my quirky spouse leaves the bathroom carpeted with his disheveled pile of pages.

After. Every. Single. Bath.

So, is it fair that when I come to take my bath, I am faced with this mess? (I can forget reading the paper myself, as reinstating it would be like a soggy MENSA challenge.) No, it isn't fair and for many years, this practice drove me up the wall. We would have 'discussions' about it and even he would agree that it wasn't fair (how could he not?). Then he would clear it up, once or twice, before lapsing into old paper-strewn habits. So, an undeniable case of the foot-stomping 'It's not fair!'s. But what to do?

Prepare to be shocked and possibly appalled: these days... *I pick up the paper and put it in the bin.* Why? Not because I feel I ought to, I don't. (And I am not yet so serene that I do it without the odd dark mutterings...) But if I leave it for him to do, it will irritate me every time I see it. Yes, it is *his* mess, but it is costing *me* in terms of negative energy.

*But that's not fair!* I hear you cry and you are absolutely right. But I *choose* to handle it this way. Within seconds, it's sorted and no longer an issue. No rows (though I may allude to it calmly but sarcastically in the future, should the opportunity arise...). And what's the worst that has happened? I've done something for someone else, something that I shouldn't have had to do. Is that really so bad? Am I so perfect that my husband doesn't occasionally have to do something on my behalf? (No, is the answer here). And what would I think of him, if he never did anything for me that was above and beyond the call of duty?

So, what's fair or what's right isn't always what's *best*. Again, not to suggest that you lie down and become a doormat or surrender to a role which is unacceptable to you. But equally, playing a victim does not serve you; it robs you of your power. So, if you can bring yourself to reject fury (at least, occasionally) you might find that it needn't be such a big deal. (Plus, if you're the type who likes to keep a mental score - they owe you one.)

Another advantage of not rising to a justified rage, and dealing with the task with serenity and calm, is the joy to be found in performing a random act of kindness - doing something for someone else that you weren't obliged to do. That way, sainthood lies.

When you opt to do kind things for other people, instead of feeling oppressed, you will feel elevated (and, if you let yourself get carried away, satisfyingly superior...). And there's more. People often notice these acts of love and care - and return them! So, in future, when you'd like a family member to do something for you (cup of tea, trip to the shop, wash car, etc), if they feel cared for and loved, they are much more likely to return the compliment. And all this in a spirit of positivity and love. Compare this to the usual tirade of 'After all I do for you, the least you can do is blah blah blah' - which may get what you want but without the bonus of family harmony and general good feelings all round.

> Being happy doesn't mean that everything is perfect.
> It means that you've decided to look beyond the imperfections.
>
> *Source unknown*

There is enough anger in the world that you can't control, but on your home territory, you have much more influence. So, why not become an example of generosity of spirit.

They say charity begins at home, but it's also a great place for peace and harmony to begin, too.

# It's a grrrl thing

As a person, it's irritating when people don't do their fair share, but if you possess any feminist tendencies, it's much more complicated. There are principles at stake. There is often the unspoken question: Is it being left to me because I am the female?

This incurs a wrath born of social inequities, turning a personal situation into a political one. It becomes less of a question about whether you should always have to clean the floor and transmutes into the much bigger issue of whether *women* should always have to clean the floor.

## Social baggage

Life is full of minor injustices. Some are gender-related, but many are not. So, in an attempt to eliminate any imagined slights, here's a suggestion: What if we dealt with each event on its own merits, without second-guessing at potential chauvinisms?

I'm the first to admit that I'm prone to taking offence at what seem to be gender-related issues. I know that I am frequently over-sensitive, reading into my husband's behaviour issues that hadn't even occurred to him. For example, I may be angrily wondering if he's left the washing up because he believes I, as the female, should do it, when in reality, he's leaving it because he simply can't be bothered. (Now *that* I can identify with....)

The feminist argument is a strong one and there are still battles to be fought, but give yourself permission, in the sanctuary of your own home, to take a little time out of the conflict.

> You don't have to be anti-man to be pro-woman.
>
> *Jane Galvin Lewis*

So instead of asking, is it fair that women have to do this, just ask, is it fair that I have to do it? The answer may still be no, but dealing with the task at hand is much less exhausting than taking on the world every time.

# Love & Marriage

Do you and your partner ever argue about housework?

It is a rare couple who don't. In survey after survey, along with money, sex, work, and children, housework features in the top five topics of domestic rows. And it's hardly surprising - what are the chances that people who live together will share perfectly aligned housework-ethics?

So, to cohabit with another person is challenging enough. However, when that other is your Significant Other, issues of love and respect can become tangled up in the domestic bickering.

Housework squabbles may be trivial on the surface, but they can do serious damage to a relationship. Any resentment that builds up around housework will undoubtedly affect your feelings towards your partner. If the resentment is founded upon a sense of injustice, the partnership loses its equality status. For any modern woman, this can lead to bitterness, anger, fury, and often the withholding of 'favours'. Hardly domestic bliss.

> Love doesn't make the world go round. Love is what makes the ride worthwhile.
>
> *Franklin P. Jones*

So, how to reinstate an equal footing and thus a more loving scenario? I have a few suggestions but before I go into those, I feel duty-bound to mention that I'm not a qualified relationships counselor. The concepts in this book are offered in the manner of well-meaning advice from a like-minded soul. My results are purely anecdotal and I can offer no guarantee that these techniques will work for you. However, if they strike a chord with you, I believe they're worth a try. (It's not always necessary to have a certificate on the wall to have something helpful to offer.) But whether advice is friendly or professional - it's always for you to decide what you will heed.

## A Triple Love Whammy.

The Beatles claimed that all you need is love, and as I am an eternal romantic, here is my three-pronged love-based solution to domestic conflict:

**1. Use the love.** In the spirit of choosing your battles wisely, it can be beneficial to air your most teeth-clenching grievances, as long as you do so in an atmosphere of mutual love and respect. Use the feelings between you as reasons to make some changes. Explain (calmly, if possible) what really bothers you, and (if you know) why. But equality works both ways, so you ought to also ask your partner what really bothers them. The results of this discussion may surprise you both. Housework is a inescapable feature of living together, so if you're committed to each other, you'll need to reach agreement on the important issues and aim for a more harmonious division of labour. Hopefully, each of you will then make the necessary efforts for the sake of your relationship, in your bid to make the one you love happy.

**2. Remember the love.** It's important to regularly step away from the battlezone and remind each other why you're together. It's very easy to get bogged down with responsibilities and the domestic workload, so aim to make regular breaks together one of your priorities. You will both be more generous and forgiving if you keep the fun and friendship levels high. Enjoy and appreciate each other again, then watch your squabbles shrink away.

**3. Apply the love.** Harsh truths: life's not fair and love's not easy. (But what are the alternatives?) All the greatest love stories involve an element of sacrifice, as do most successful relationships. Admittedly, cooking when it's his turn is not quite in the same league as drinking poison, but the principle is the same - the things you do for love. Saying 'I love you' is easy; more difficult is *proving it*. But this is what you're being asked to do in those moments that require compromise or tolerance, when you dig deep into your heart and do things out of love. This may not be easy, but then, who said it was going to be? As a consolation, the subsequent rewards will make your sacrifice worthwhile. Love is like a boomerang. It can go a long way but it always comes back to you.

> Marrying is easy, it's housework that's hard.
>
> *Proverb*

## No complaints

More in the spirit of harmony than justice (though one often follows the other), this is a useful tip on what *not* to do: complain. I can almost hear those splutters of protest, but bear with me. Firstly, it does no good. It's ineffective. Actually it's worse, it's *counter*productive. Secondly, it can truly do harm to your relationship. Thirdly, it's bad for your health. A life of complaining - *however justified* - will only give you wrinkles or gallstones or worse, as well as more to complain about.

So, unless a cycle of resentment and ill-health works for you, make a decision to halt it. It will be tough at first (and you may need to find other avenues to vent your frustration) but it will get easier, and the results will be worth it. You will have more inner and outer peace. I promise.

## Lead by example

One final idea, which is a bit of a wild card but if times are desperate, it may be worth a try.

I nagged and berated my husband for years, to no avail. I cannot think of a single occasion when any of my haranguing achieved the desired result. Then one day, out of sheer desperation, I caved. I cleaned up *his* mess - and a miracle happened! After seeing me do this for him, without a word between us, he started to pick up his clothes. He washed up more. He even vacuumed. I was so shocked that it could be so simple that I tried it again, and again. And it worked!

> Love is saying 'I feel differently' instead of 'You're wrong'.
>
> *Anon.*

Whether it was passive-aggressive, guilt, or some skewed competitive streak, I neither know nor care. It was a route to my happy outcome without a single raised voice. It took me years, YEARS! to learn this lesson. I think we can safely call that learning the hard way.

So, why not try it? What's the worst that could happen – you end up with a tidier home (and probably a stronger marriage)?

# Why, oh why?

Solutions to problems needn't always involve a change in circumstances.

If you feel more incensed by other's behaviour when you simply cannot comprehend it, if you ever find yourself venting exasperated cries of, *Why do they do this?* or *Why don't they do that?* or *I just can't understand it!* - one answer could simply be *increased understanding.*

Very often, it's the sense of confusion surrounding the offence that causes the most irritation. Our brains like answers. They're programmed to keep puzzling over a question until it makes sense. So if the Others do something that not only annoys you but also baffles you, the incident will hang around for longer in your head, quietly sapping your mental energy in a search for an explanation.

In our mission to increase your domestic harmony and mental peace, it's time to throw a soupçon of understanding into the mix. To do this, you need to temporarily let go of your take on an issue and try to see it from *their side.*

If you can unearth the thinking behind their behaviour, it can lead to a surprisingly satisfying 'Aha!' moment: So *that's* why!

When you can understand an offence, even though it may still be unjustified, *it will irritate you so much less.* In striving for understanding, *you* will benefit - you'll find it easier to cope with the issue and will deal with it more calmly.

Doesn't that sound more appealing than the baffled and bewildered fury?

## Have you ever...

In my bid to understand my family's behaviour, I like to play a little mental game called 'Have I ever...' Here are the rules:

Think of a reoccurring offence within your household that really baffles you. For example, I get het up with confused frustration by my family's inability to hang up wet towels. I've explained to them that it's not merely a personal preference, but that a second's effort can make the difference between a towel ready for another use and a smelly damp pile of unnecessary laundry. So, if they carelessly opt to create more washing (for me) - I am not a happy bunny. Since I have explained the logic to them, it baffles me - why don't they just *hang up the (bleep, bleep) towel?!*

So far, so understandable (and familiar?), right? Well, here's where my little game comes in. I am generally in the habit of hanging up wet towels but if I ask: Have I *ever* left one on the floor/bed/chair?, if I am honest, my answer is, yes I have. Not very often (and always with good reason, of course) but I have done it.

So, if I have *ever* done it, even if only once, I can *understand* how easily it can be done. I can see how it might happen, without any deliberate inconsideration or malice. In which case, maybe, just maybe, the Others had good reasons, too. Perhaps, they didn't do it out of a lack of regard for me and my laundry levels, after all. They just didn't hang up the towel.

When you can understand others' behaviour, it may still be annoying, but it's no longer baffling. If even *you* can commit the 'offence', it's *understandable*. You may be surprised by the effect this subtle difference can have.

## Just imagine...

Here's another little game for dealing with an acute sense of down-troddenness.*

When you leap to the conclusion that you're being intentionally treated unfairly by someone, you're assuming a certain thought process on their behalf. Now, in some cases you may be right, but *even if you are right* - this trick can help to relieve some of your frustration.

So let's play 'Just Imagine'. Can you imagine a different scenario, one where you are not being victimised? Is it at all possible that they have a different agenda than treating you unfairly? Perhaps they left out the breakfast things not because they view it as your job but because they were running late. The consequences for you may not even have entered their head. (This may lead you to conclude that they are inconsiderate, but at least they're not oppressing you.)

If you are going to imagine the preceding course of events or train of thought - *opt for the version that gives you the most peace.*

---

*Quick tip: making up games is good. If you can inject an element of fun into a problem, the benefits can be twofold. Firstly, a light-hearted approach is often more likely to yield a satisfactory solution. Secondly, playing is good for you. Domestic life can be tough - grab a little light relief when and where you can!

It might even be the right one! But even if you give them credit for being nicer than they actually are, does it really matter? Who knows, they just might start living up to your elevated view of them. Not a bad side effect.

So practice imagining alternative scenarios to the one that leaves you seething. You cannot see into their heads, so give them the benefit of any doubt. You may or may not be letting them off the hook, but either way, it reduces your stress-levels. So you will actually be doing the biggest favour to yourself.

## What you see is what you get

In the fascinating world of neuroscience (stay with me), the clever folk are coming up with amazing discoveries about how our brains work. I like to take these (the ones I can understand...) and twist them to my own end, i.e., use them to, if not solve, then at least explain certain aspects of the Housework Blues.

One of these is the concept of *brain filters* - in other words, what we 'see' (as referred to briefly on page 37).

Many years into my marriage I made a remarkable discovery about my husband - he just doesn't *see* what I see. Previously, I would silently fume over a mess he'd ignored, or if I confronted him with it – he'd appear genuinely surprised to have it pointed out. It's impossible, I'd say, *to not see it* - it's right there! Impossible! Or was it...?

Time for the science bit...

We see with our eyes, right? Wrong. We see *through* our eyes. Millions of pieces of information enter our vision *every second*. Millions! We don't see, or notice, all of these on a conscious level, otherwise our brains would short-circuit. We are only aware of a fraction of this bombardment (maybe as little as 1%).

So who or what decides which bits we actually notice? Not our eyes - but our brain, whose job it is to determine what's *relevant to us* and disregard the rest. That's why no two people will view the same scene the same way - because everyone's brain will filter according to their individual criteria.

Our criteria are dictated by our beliefs and experiences, amassed over our lifetime and unique to us. It's our personal perspective, our individual view.

Allow me to illustrate this with an example. I once called at the home of a neighbour, whom I didn't know very well. I hadn't expected to be invited in, but when I was, I was bowled over by the exquisite interior - slate floors, stripped pine, luxuriant soft furnishings - it was like something from an interiors magazine. I made several gushing remarks about her home (I struggled to hide my awe) but my neighbour looked mortified! She said things like, 'Oh, the floor needs cleaning! I've been meaning to do it... Just look at it! It's filthy! Oh, I'm so embarrassed!'

Now I was only in the house for a matter of minutes - it's unlikely I would have noticed whether her floor needed cleaning and since I wasn't planning to eat my dinner off it, it wasn't an issue...for me. When I looked at my neighbour's floor, I saw beautiful Indian slate, but she looked at it and saw a job she'd failed to do. That's brain filters at work. Our personal perspective plays a huge part in what we 'see'.

*Perception is a mirror, not a fact.*

*A Course in Miracles*

Applied to the home front, when it comes to those minor chores - some people will see them and some (lucky them!), won't. For example, think of all the niggling jobs in your own home - they're undeniably annoying, right? But does your entire household feel the same way? Do your children stress over their unmade beds? Does your partner lose sleep over the clutter levels? My guess is, no - it's just you. But why? Those jobs exist, there's no rule to say they're purely your problem, so why is it just you who is fretting about them?

You may feel that it's unfair that they leave certain jobs to you, but could it be a matter of differing perspectives? Perhaps, they haven't consciously left it for you...they just haven't noticed it at all! And in the spirit of justice, is it *fair* to blame your housemates for what they simply don't see?

So if we accept all this, what then can we do about it? Well, the good news is that brain filters are not set in stone. They can be changed, through effort and repetition. It is possible to train the brain and influence what you (or they) notice and to what you remain oblivious. (So, if you can't beat 'em, you could always join 'em!) Persistently pointing out to your housemates what needs doing, should eventually get through to them - but this is not the easiest or most harmonious use of this information.

There's an alternative, more enlightened way to view the problem. Firstly, resolve that *you* will handle the jobs that *you* notice. (You can't be expected to deal with jobs you haven't noticed, but equally, neither can your family.) And armed with your newfound understanding as to why the Others haven't done them, you'll be less annoyed and feel less exploited. (In theory, at least.)

Secondly, acknowledge that it's likely (or at least possible) that they may see jobs that you don't! For example, my husband is constantly berating me for neglecting my car maintenance. I even agree with him that it's a potential safety hazard, but those are just not jobs that crop up on my radar. So he very kindly deals with them. This makes me more inclined to deal with the jobs of which he lives in blissful ignorance. This creates a happy scenario where we each go with, rather than against, the flow.

Now this system may not divide the workload into precisely equal parts (particularly if you have a tendency to keep score) but at least it tips those scales of justice in the right direction. There's some comfort in knowing that as you're picking up the slack for others, they may well be doing the same for you. You move the atmosphere from one of injustice and oppression to one of mutual support.

Keeping this in mind will not only result in less resentment in your heart, but also a healthier atmosphere of give and take in your home. Which is a pretty fair return.

> We don't see things as they are, we see things as we are.
>
> *Anais Nin*

# To err is human...

...to forgive is divine.

In this sense, I use 'divine' as in related to higher powers, rather than wonderful fun. For me, at least, forgiveness does not always come easily. But there's a saying that nothing worthwhile is easy. And an ability, or even just an intention, to practice more forgiveness is an effort which will reap unbelievable benefits.

## Why forgive?

Within the self-help genre, a ubiquitous tip to moving towards peace, health, even wealth, is to let go of grievances. What the experts in this field know is that blame, however justified, hurts *you*. So in addition to the wrong you have suffered, if you harbour a grudge, you are exposing yourself to further damage. It costs you in terms of mental and emotional energy and, more seriously, in terms of your health.

Perhaps the most recent application of this theory is through the previously-mentioned Emotional Freedom Techniques (EFT). This practice is based on the belief that emotions are the root cause of all physical ailments. The idea is that any imbalance in the body is directly related to a blockage in our body's energy system - caused by our negative emotions. The ramifications of this are significant - emotions such as resentment and bitterness can literally make you ill.

> Before you begin on the journey of revenge, dig two graves.
>
> *Proverb*

Even beyond the relatively new science of EFT, examples abound of people who decide to put a past wrong behind them and find that their seemingly unrelated ailments miraculously vanish. The Sedona Method, as already mentioned, is also a highly regarded system that supports this philosophy. And Catherine Ponder's book, *The Dynamic Laws of Prosperity*, is full of stories that suggest a link between bearing a grudge and physical ailments. She writes, 'If you are now in a state of ill-health, there is something, somebody or some memory you need to forgive and release from your feelings forever.'

It would seem, then, that forgiveness is not only virtuous, but good for you, too.

## So what's stopping us?

Considering we're known as the gentler sex, women do sometimes have a penchant for wielding, rather than burying, the hatchet. Maybe it's down to our psychological or hormonal make-up, but women are notorious for stewing over wrongs for much longer than our menfolk. In my own experience, my husband is often amazed that I can still be smarting over a comment made three days previously.

But we are emotional beings, even if to varying degrees, and as such tend to take things to heart. To forgive and forget may be sage advice, but it often goes against our natural instincts. (But then men have issues like male pride to keep them simmering, so maybe life is not so unjust after all...)

Regardless of the whys and wherefores of our grievances, though, reducing or eliminating them is in *our best interests*. If you strive for more harmony in your home and serenity in your head, then forgiveness is one great way to go. Hopefully

> Hell hath no fury like a woman scorned.
>
> *William Congreve*

some of the suggestions within this book will make you better placed to naturally forgive - understanding more and judging less can be powerful techniques and hugely beneficial. But if, like me, knowing what you should do doesn't always help you to do it, here are some further tips to smooth the rocky road to forgiveness.

**Acknowledge.** Don't try to deny your feelings. Suppression is not the same as forgiveness and can lead to more serious consequences. You may, after all, be harbouring legitimate resentments. So express or air your objections if you really need to, but try to do this as a means to moving on, rather than a habit of dwelling on the issue. Before you can put your grievances behind you, you may need to face up to them and deal with them. But this is preferable to the low-level brooding, which only harms you in the long run.

**Practice.** Like most things, forgiving gets easier with practice. So, if at first you don't succeed... don't worry! Just try again the next time. And if you are feeling too utterly resentful towards the guilty party to forgive them, it may help to remember that you're doing it for *you*, not them.

**Don't give up.** It is human nature to want to blame - so if that's your first instinct: forgive yourself! You're only human. It does not mean that you can't do the forgiveness thing. It will take time before it becomes an easy reaction for you. In fact, it will be an ongoing attitude, a lifelong intention, rather than an end result.

**Leave it to karma.** If your sense of justice is too finely tuned to just let it go, have faith in karma. If you believe that there are forces at work that even the score, and that you don't need to be the one to administer retribution, you will find it much easier to get past any slights or offences. (I tend not to invoke this method towards my loved ones, but beyond the home, I have a phrase that helps me walk away from people who have wronged me: *What goes around comes around.* Admittedly it's not the most charitable sentiment – but if you have an acute sense of justice, it can help you keep your cool.)

I have always found that mercy bears richer fruits than strict justice.

*Abraham Lincoln*

**Soul-search.** It may often be the case that you are rightfully indignant and under no reasonable obligation to forgive. But have you ever been on the other side of such a scenario? There may come a time when you are in the wrong and hoping for forgiveness. People make mistakes, possibly you (and most definitely me), included. I find that asking, *Am I perfect?* sometimes helps me overlook the shortcomings of others, (since I know the answer to be a resounding *No!*).

Q: Why should I…?

A: Why shouldn't you?

# Take 100% responsibility

Who is responsible for where you are right now?

It's often tempting to feel that other people or external circumstances are mostly to blame, that we are being buffeted and tossed by the fickle seas of fate and destiny.

If you feel this way, prepare yourself for a difficult but ultimately empowering revelation: You are accountable for your own life.

Whilst it's true that you can't command every aspect of your life, you are where you are in your life, right at this moment, because of a multitude of decisions and choices, both major and trivial, all made by *you*. You may not be able to dictate what life throws at you, but you are in absolute control of your reaction to it. This is your power.

*The willingness to accept responsibility for one's own life is the source from which self-respect springs.*

*Joan Didion*

In recognizing this, don't be tempted to begin blaming yourself for any current woes - blame is a useless activity, and self-blame can be incredibly destructive. So look forward, not back. See this as a call to recognize and seize your power to improve your current situation. You're only a victim if you accept that role, and in doing so you would be ignoring the formidable forces within that can shape your life and your destiny.

Taking responsibility for your life might not be pleasant. It may be easier to think we have no choice - but how is that belief serving you? Accepting that you are accountable for your own life is a vital step in bringing about the changes you would like to see, not just in household issues, but across every aspect of your life. Now is the time to stop blaming others, acknowledge where you are, where you want to be, and what you're going to do about it. You do have options. There is always a choice.

This particular insight hit home to me when I was on my hands and knees scrubbing the kitchen floor, feeling very disillusioned with my lot. I was cross and disappointed that 'this was my life'. Then, like a slap across my sulky face, I was struck with the realisation that *I* was responsible. My circumstances in that moment were a culmination of a lifetime's worth of decisions that I had freely made. It was no one else's fault - it was down to me.

Of course, then I began to ask where had I gone wrong... but gradually I wondered, had I really gone wrong at all? Hadn't I always chosen the routes I wanted to take, taking on a home, a family. Were these mistakes? Or was cleaning the floor just part of the package that I had *voluntarily* signed up for? It was my own life choices that meant I had a floor to clean, and actually, I didn't regret them.

As a result of this new perspective, I began to think that having a home is actually a blessing, and having to maintain it was a small price - which I was suddenly very happy and willing to pay. The resentment and frustration left me. I began to relax. I was still on my hands and knees cleaning a floor - on the outside, nothing had changed - but after my internal epiphany, I'd gone from feeling miserable and downtrodden to feeling grateful and lucky. (I'd have felt luckier still if a maid had been due, but still, one step at a time...).

> When you blame others, you give up your power to change.
>
> Author Unknown

This may have been a subtle internal shift - owning my fate - but the relief, calm and new sense of contentedness were significant.

Once you make the (albeit difficult) decision to not be a victim of circumstances, your whole attitude changes. You leave the blaming and complaining behind (where did they ever get you?). This alone is enormously liberating (and good for you!). Though it can be a little scary to realise that your life is in your own hands, it can also be an exhilarating rush of potential and possibility. Accepting 100% responsibility enables you to look to the future with optimism and hope.

Taking this step will unleash powerful forces within you that may have so far been dormant. You may feel like you can take on the world! And in this spirit of empowerment and world domination - your domestic gripes will rapidly diminish. You may even find they vanish altogether.

# The long straws

Do you ever feel that you're always getting the raw deal, the messy end of the stick, the short straw? Have you ever grumbled, *It's alright for them...*? Do you sometimes indulge in a 'Woe is me' moment?

If you answered yes to any of the above, it could be time to look for the long straws.

## Raindrops on roses

Time to go from the sobs of self-pity to *The Sound of Music*... and think of a few of your favourite things! Think of the things in your life that make you feel good, that you feel fortunate to experience. Call to mind the best bits about being you. Just stop for a moment and try it. No, really, do it now....

Found something? Excellent! That's your long straw. These are the rewards you get in this bargain you've struck with life. We often get so wound up about what's not working, we forget to notice what is. So it can be reassuring to recall these blessings, to redress the balance if you feel that the world is against you.

This exercise works on two levels. Firstly, the fact that you can't focus on two things simultaneously means that by considering the nicer aspects of your life, you automatically stop dwelling on the negatives. This alone will relieve a good deal of your angst.

Secondly, when you turn your attention to your long straws, you magically feel less resentful of the downsides. It's hard to feel badly-done-to when you begin cataloguing all the wonderful things you have. As a result, your attitude shifts, and you go from down to up.

Allow me to illustrate with a personal example. When I was housebound with a new baby, I would become enraged that my husband could casually nip into the golf club as the whim struck, whereas I had to plan my outings like a military operation. 'It's just not fair!' I would stomp and pout, focussing on my short straw - the temporary restriction. But after a concerted effort, I began to acknowledge certain advantages to my stay-at-home routine - coffee with a friend, a spot of gardening, pram-pushing on a sunny day, leisurely breakfasts as my husband would rush off to an early meeting.

These were my long straws which I had begun to take for granted.

In considering them, I was forced to admit that my life wasn't so bad, after all. It was quite a humbling experience and one that put paid to any stroppy resentments.

Acknowledging the plus-sides put the occasional downsides into perspective and made them much easier to bear. In fact, it turned out that my husband actually considered me to be the one who had it easy! Perhaps you and your partner have had similar 'discussions'. Many of us have a tendency to believe we are the most unfortunate. But instead of competing for who's getting the worst deal, we'd all be better off if we shifted the focus away from the flaws and towards the fabulous.

Once you start this process, you may be pleasantly surprised at how many long straws you can think of. Happily, the rule of 'whatever you focus on expands' applies to the good stuff just as much as the dross. Simply by seeking out your 'diamonds in the dust-heap', you'll unearth more and more of them.

So the next time you're enjoying yourself, doing something you love, whatever that may be, register it as a long straw. Acknowledge that you have that good in your life. And don't forget, whenever you come across these joys, give yourself a pat on the back. If you're going to take responsibility for whatever is going wrong, you also get to take credit for anything you're doing right! So, if you have manoeuvred your life to include these little snippets of pleasure, delight in that too.

The more regularly you seek and find your long straws, the more ammunition you'll have when your woes threaten to send you into a downward spiral. But happily, when the attitude of counting your blessings becomes automatic, you'll find fewer occasions when you need to use it to fend off the blues.

> Count your
> blessings.
>
> *Proverb*

# Write your own job description...

Now here's a contentious issue – what is a woman's work? Or a wife's? Or a mother's?

Since the advent of feminism, women have been raised to believe that they have more to offer than *merely* caring for a family. Whilst it's true that women have potential beyond the home, there's an implication that caring for a family is an inferior choice or a waste of talents, or even a denial of your sense of self.

With the blurring of social boundaries in recent years, the world's expectations of a woman/wife/mother have been radically and irrevocably altered. Whilst the pursuit of equality is undoubtedly the right path, a side effect of our new options is a generation of women who are unsure of what is acceptable and expected. Many of us wonder how our domestic demands fit in with our new freedoms. Can you be a feminist and a housewife? How much cooking and cleaning should a modern liberated woman be doing?

On a personal note, I opted for a home and a family; in fact, it was my dream (at least, part of it). Yet I have a strong sense of equality and a degree of ambition. So when it comes to the maintenance of my home and family, I have been known to grumble, *I shouldn't be doing this...should I?*

Ultimately, the right role for any woman is the one she takes on willingly and happily, regardless of social dictates. All women are different, so naturally, our views on domestic obligations will vary. Determining which of the chores justly fall to you is completely your call. You know better than anyone what you feel is right.

But actually taking this step - specifying what is acceptable (to you) - can be a useful exercise in dealing with feelings of injustice.

## Clarify your terms

You may bemoan the unfairness of having to do work that isn't 'your job'. But are you as swift to admit what you *are* responsible for?

Have you even really considered this? If not, take the time to set down, in black and white, those jobs that you feel could be reasonably assigned to you. In your role within the home, which jobs will you willingly accept responsibility for? Keeping a home is an occupation and as such needs distinct guidelines as to what is and isn't within your realm of accountability. So to clear up any issues of what you should or shouldn't be doing, take the time to write your own job description.

As you do this, however, bear in mind your keenness for justice! So be fair. For example, if you chose to have children, you are at least partly liable for the ensuing upkeep and care. Or if you were the one who opted for a large home, who do you feel is responsible for its maintenance?

Clarifying what falls within your jurisdiction can be useful in two ways. Firstly, the jobs which make it onto your self-penned contract, you can then do without resentment. It's likely that some of the jobs we moan about haven't *unjustly fallen to us*, it's simply that we don't want to do them. Realising this relieves any mental angst over whether you are being taken advantage of. If you have voluntarily agreed your terms, there is less inclination (or justification) to complain. There is even a certain pride at stake, and honour to be found in rising to your self-selected challenges.

Secondly, you identify the jobs that you begrudge, the ones you feel aren't rightfully down to you. These are the chores that cause resentment to build up, so it can be helpful to suss out them out.

> Not only is women's work never done, the definition keeps changing.
>
> *Bill Copeland*

These aren't necessarily the most unpleasant jobs. You may readily agree that some horrid tasks are down to you. For example, if my child vomits - who, on the entire planet, is the person most liable for the cleaning-up? It's not a joyful task, but I accept that it's down to me.

The problem-chores are the ones that you feel you shouldn't be doing, when you sense, deep down, that something has gone wrong. These are the ones that make you dwell on thoughts of injustice. Once you identify these, the easiest solution would be simply to delegate them (either within the home or without). However, delegation is not always an option. So if you must deal with chores that cause you disproportionate angst, fury or resentment, try to discover the root cause of your objection. Often when you understand why you feel so strongly, it becomes clear how to deal with the problem. Simply identifying the underlying issue may be enough to defuse the matter.

Whatever you have to do in order to come to terms with the jobs you strongly object to will be worthwhile. Denying or ignoring your feelings and pretending you can cope won't work in the long term. It will only result in a simmering resentment which will, eventually, erupt (and that probably won't be pretty...) By hauling these issues into the light, you can then begin dealing with them.

So, taking these two steps - clarifying what you are happy to take on, and dealing with whatever is not acceptable - will eliminate many of those vague feelings of 'Why should I?' When you define your responsibilities, you will feel more in control and less exploited. Although your workload may not differ greatly, when you know a particular job is within your agreed job description, you can at least ditch those unpleasant feelings of oppression.

## Fair or reasonable?

Before you embark on deciding what is rightfully down to you, I'd like to make a distinction: It's not necessary to accept only what is absolutely fair. There is room for elements of voluntary giving, charitable acts, kindness, nurturing, etc, especially within a home full of people you love.

For example, is it fair that I always cook my children's meals? They never cook mine! Technically, that's an injustice but trying to settle that score would be childish (and futile). So, perhaps in writing your job description, instead of asking is it fair, ask: Is it reasonable? It's OK (and admirable) to include jobs that you aren't obliged to do, but that you want to do, whether out of a sense of duty or the goodness of your kind and generous heart.

## Duty calls

Duty. Now, there's a loaded word. It's a brave partner/child/other who would argue that you should perform a task because *it is your duty*. Our predecessors have (mostly) banished dated ideas of subjugated females being 'rightfully' chained to the kitchen sink. But just because it is no longer politically correct to cite a woman's duty as keeping a home, does that mean we're relieved of all duties with regard to partners and children, family and friends, even to ourselves? In rejecting the stereotypical woman's work, keen to assure the world what is not our duty, are we as keen to determine what *is*?

To speak of a woman's duty today is often regarded as sexist, but if we pause in our knee-jerk reaction, duty has many admirable connotations: responsibility, obligation, commitment, allegiance, loyalty, faithfulness, fidelity, homage. It is related to honour and our contribution to the world. When a man does his duty, it is respectable, praiseworthy and impressive. For true equality between the sexes, then, women would also see duty as a positive and embrace it. If we make our own commitments, accept our own responsibilities and determine for ourselves what our duties will be, there is no shame in admitting to duties in our lives.

For example, I am married and I accept that I have duties as a wife. Now, before you think I've gone soft, let me assure you that it will be a cold day in hell before I'll concede that those duties directly include *all* the cooking and cleaning. However, I will accept that in my (voluntary) commitment to my husband, I took on responsibilities to support and care for him. Isn't that what marriage is all about?

> All the great things are simple, and many can be expressed in a single word: freedom, justice, honor, duty, mercy, hope.
>
> *Winston Churchill*

Of course, I expect it to run both ways. It's an equal relationship, but it is also mutually nurturing - the typical 'I scratch your back and you scratch mine' scenario.

The problems tend to arise when one of us thinks we're doing an unfair share of the scratching. If the situation occurs where you're the only one doing your duty, arguably, that's not fair. But does that mean you should stop doing your duty....or the other party should start?

## Take on jobs of honour

Coming to terms with your responsibility is good for your self esteem. Once you have agreed, accepted and embraced your duty, it is empowering to know that you're meeting your commitments out of a sense of honour, and not because someone else has dictated your circumstances. To utilise some of this motivation, attach the idea of honour to certain jobs within your home. You can do this either for the jobs you loathe but know you should do or those jobs that will have the most (positive) impact on those you love/live with.

For example, I like to ensure, as my personal responsibility, that there are always supplies of milk and bread in the house. This may seem a trivial task but it is a key element to the smooth running of my family - and as wife, mother, and lady of the house, that's something I feel duty-bound, and happy, to take on.

So see if you can assign your own jobs of honour. Start with the small things, if necessary, but try to get past any socio-political pressures. Then, as you embrace these *voluntary* commitments to your family, you'll naturally reduce any simmering resentments.

Which has got to be a good thing – not least for you.

# ...but don't be a jobsworth.

Although defining acceptable roles can be helpful, be prepared for an element of flexibility. The aim isn't to become a Jobsworth - someone who is a stickler for the contract, doing the bare minimum and nothing more. Besides, there are tremendous benefits to going above and beyond the call of duty, and not only for those on the receiving end of your generosity. Being willing to do more than your fair share can be a gratifying and auspicious way to live.

## Motherly love

When you are ill, or down, or heartbroken - who would you choose to look after you? I, like most people I know, turn to that antithesis of the Jobsworth: my mum. During the lows of life, a bit of maternal pampering is what you need, someone who not only meets your needs, but anticipates and exceeds them. Most of us can remember a feeling of being totally and lovingly cared for - and wasn't it lovely?

Well, it's within your power to reproduce that warm and happy feeling in those you love. Whether you're a mother or not, that caring instinct is present in all women (admittedly in varying degrees...) and it is something to be valued, cherished and encouraged. Curiously, and wonderfully, these kind-hearted acts often reward the giver as much as the recipient.

## The extra mile

Have you ever come across a person or service that adequately met your needs - but nothing more? Compare that to a time when somebody did something extra, and provided more than was necessary. Maybe it was just a small gesture, an offer of help, a smile. Or perhaps you've been in a restaurant, hotel or shop, where the service was above and beyond what was expected. How did those little extras make you feel? They probably cheered you up. They may even have made your day.

Can you imagine the increase in peace and harmony in the world if everyone sought to create that feeling in others? Well, your home is a small but significant place to start. Let's face it - most homes are just bursting with opportunities to go the extra mile! So it is well within your power to make a difference in the world, just by doing those little extras for your family.

## What's in it for you?

To go above and beyond your obligations is not only admirable, it's also rewarding. Consider the restaurateur, the hotelier or shopkeeper who went above and beyond the call of duty - what did they get for their efforts? It's possible they received nothing more than your admiration and gratitude. But how do we feel when people admire and appreciate us? We feel great!

> Those who bring sunshine into the lives of others, cannot keep it from themselves.
>
> *J M Barrie*

So their efforts for others bring *them* good feelings. It's also very likely that their generosity will also bring them repeat business. It's a win-win.

However... the rewards may not always be in the form of recognition or thanks - and if you expect those, you could be disappointed. You may get them, but you may not. You may never know whether your work has even been noticed. But there is goodness in the gesture, not just the result. The magic occurs within you. It's good for your soul. It's also good for your sense of self - who doesn't want to regard themselves as good and kind and caring?

So try to cultivate an attitude of doing more than is justly required. Do it solely for the joy in knowing that you're spreading a little happiness. And if you believe in karma, you can rest easy in the knowledge that your random acts of kindness will come back to you.

Whilst it's true that, for peace of mind, it's good to be clear about your obligations, for peace of heart, it's good to go above and beyond them. As often as you like.

# Service with a smile

If you feel an injustice in your domestic life, it may be there is a gap (chasm?) between what you do willingly and what is being left for 'someone' to do.

One solution is to encourage your housemates to do more (and good luck with that...). But it may also help to look at the problem from the opposite side, i.e., how you feel about your obligations. If you could, somehow, become *naturally inclined to do more for your family* - voluntarily - you would feel less resentful and put upon.

So, let's look at how to encourage that, but before we do, let's first consider if that's the right thing to do. Is it a backward step for feminism to seek to serve more? Is it demeaning to shoulder more of the burden? For modern women, there is a worry that serving is not compatible with a sense of dignity and equality. There is also the more universal concern that in becoming more subservient, we will be disrespected or exploited.

Is it possible to serve without being a doormat?

## Service as weakness?

Mother Teresa is perhaps the most perfect example, in recent times, of a life dedicated to service. And how does the world feel about her? She is universally admired and respected. Far from making her inferior to the rest of us, her life of selfless attendance to the needs of others is highly regarded and esteemed. For some she is seen as a modern-day saint. I, for one, feel very humbled and unworthy when I think of people like Mother Teresa, who give of themselves so selflessly.

Many of the world's religious, spiritual or political leaders, *figures that the world looks up to*, also achieved greatness through their service to others. The Buddha believed that to be happy, you serve others; to be miserable, you serve yourself. Albert Einstein claimed that the high destiny of the individual is to serve rather than to rule. Jesus Christ famously washed the feet of his apostles - the ultimate subservient act.

Admittedly, it can be tough to overcome the psychology of being the server. Humans can be naturally selfish, more inclined to be on the receiving end of service, the one being served. But, as perverse and illogical as it seems, in serving others, *you* are rewarded. In business, for example, the provision of quality service is a fundamental ingredient of success, and subsequently, financial reward.

It would appear, then, that a willingness to serve can be a strength. However, womankind has only just shaken off the shackles of enforced servitude. It's tempting for feminists to view service as a kind of weakness, an inequality, an old oppression to be avoided. But the essential difference here is in *electing* to serve. Voluntary service is not enslavement. We're not being exploited if we choose to do it.

Perhaps, then, within our own homes, we could view service not as a feminist issue, but a human issue, less about playing the good housewife, than being a good person. Instead of indignantly rejecting the notion of women's work, we could use our uniquely female capabilities to improve not only our own lives, but those of the people we care about.

> The secret of being happy is doing things for other people.
>
> Dick Gregory

Mahatma Gandhi claimed that we all render services, consciously or not, but if we could do it *deliberately*, our desire for service would grow - to our own benefit and the rest of the world.

Domestic life can be a never-ending cycle of work. If we can, at least some of the time, develop an attitude of willingness to serve - like that smiling hotelier - it might actually lead to more joy in our own hearts. And as a result, we'll create more peace within our homes and, by extension, the world at large.

Quite a result, for the 'weaker sex'.

# It's for you!

Why do we do all that we do? *Who* are we doing it for?

## Take a day off!

Here's a fun tip which will shed some light on your hidden agenda. Just for a day, impose a housework ban. Step away from the vacuum cleaner. The duster is out of bounds. Washing, ironing, cooking, cleaning - all off. Do not tidy up. For one day only, do absolutely nothing. (Don't worry, your home and family won't fall apart after just one day, though you may need to dine out...)

Now, this may seem perverse advice in a book about conquering housework, but it is surprisingly effective. This exercise will (hopefully) highlight to you just how much you actually *want* to take care of your home. Yes, the sheer volume of work may get you down, the repetitive nature, the thankless, invisible chores. But by restraining yourself from dealing with it, you'll see that not doing it isn't such a great alternative.

By the end of the day, if you manage to get that far, you will be itching to get back to work. It's a basic human instinct to care for our homes, to spend time and attention keeping them comfortable and clean. We naturally seek order and tidiness. So it can be difficult to see our domain descend into squalor and chaos without intervening. (Admittedly, this instinct is perhaps more honed in the female of the species.)

So what do we learn from this? That much of the wonderful work you do is... because you want to! It's a labour of love. It's true that, indirectly, you may be doing it for your family but, in essence you are doing it for you. You want to look after your home and who can blame you? We all have to live somewhere - given the choice, who wouldn't opt for a more pleasant and agreeable environment?

It can be a relief to learn that what you are doing is through choice, rather than begrudging circumstances. Knowing this, you can then approach housework more positively - not because you have to, but because you prefer order to chaos, cleanliness to grubbiness and grime.

A bonus side effect of this experiment is its effect on your housemates. Inform them of your intention in advance, so they don't inflict their demands on you during your day of domestic exile. Then stick to the plan. All-out strikes are very effective - it's amazing how quickly you will be surrounded by dirty pots and dirty clothes, empty wardrobes and empty tummies. Your family will soon begin to notice all the invisible work you do - *when it doesn't get done*. After one day of fending for themselves, they should have a renewed respect for all your hard work. (At least for a day or so...)

## Taking care of No. 1

We tend to hold our families responsible for our workload - and undoubtedly they do add to it - but if you lived alone, there would still be housework.

Even if we only had ourselves to look after, there's still a significant degree of maintenance involved. Much of the work we do for the whole family, we would do anyway, for ourselves. We will always need to buy food and plan meals and cook them and wash up.

Also the domestic schedule doesn't always increase in proportion to the number of people living in one place. For example, cooking for two doesn't take twice as long as cooking for one. Cleaning a shared space wouldn't be any quicker if only you lived there. And dust will gather regardless of occupancy.

So, when you're feeling the strain of caring for other people, it can be helpful to remember that you'd have to do a significant amount of your workload anyway - purely for yourself. In reality, how much extra work do those you love/live with actually add? Undoubtedly, there are areas where they do create more work (laundry, for example). But, hopefully, when you call to mind the reason you have these people in your home, you'll decide they're worth the extra effort.

## Essential or preference?

Here's one final thing to consider, in our pursuit of justice. When you complain about your family not doing their fair share - do you mean a reasonable share of *essential* work?

For example, is the workload dictated by what is necessary for health and hygiene? Or is it simply what *you* would prefer to be done? How much of what you expect of them is to meet *your* version of what's necessary?

Let's say your teenage son is quite happy with an unmade bed. He does have logic on his side - it will only get unmade again at bedtime. You may argue that it's *nicer* when it's made. But nicer for whom? If he doesn't care, should he do it just to please you? (You may feel that yes, he should, but I can offer no solution for that reasoning in a section about injustice.)

So before you claim that your family aren't doing what's expected, ask yourself, is 'what's expected' a reasonable contribution? Or could it be more what *you* deem to be a decent effort to meet your exacting standards?

In the interests of justice - are your demands a fair expectation?

# Section 3:

# futility

# What's the point?

If you think too much about housework, the utter futility of it could drive you mad.

It's an endeavour that can never be fully completed. Any progress will inevitably be undone, often before your very eyes and usually by the people you love! Little wonder housework gets under our skin - it comes close to the definition of psychological torment.

## Threading beads on a string with no knot

Simone de Beauvoir likened housework to the torture of Sisyphus - a character from Greek mythology who, as punishment for cheating death, was condemned to pushing a boulder up a mountain, only to have it always roll to the bottom before it ever reached the top. The gods could think of no worse punishment for him than to be damned to an eternity of futile and hopeless labor - endless physical effort combined with the mental torment of the pointlessness of it all. Sound familiar?

Housework is a never-ending cycle. You clean, it gets dirty, so you clean again. You cook, it gets eaten, so you cook again, ad infinitum... But isn't that also the nature of life? You wake, eat, work, play (if you're lucky), then sleep. Day after day after day.

> In order for something to become clean, something else must become dirty.
>
> *Imbesi's Conservation of Filth Law*

If we look too closely at this we could get lost in the mists of existential angst - which has pushed many a great mind over the edge. So, how do we come to terms with the issue of futility without resorting to the despairing cry of, *What's it all for?*

Greater minds than mine have pondered these issues. In fact entire religions and philosophies have been borne from such musings. Some have, helpfully, come up with a few ideas on how to deal with the problem (and stay sane). I have distilled, interpreted, twisted and added to some of these and offer them to you now - to assist you in pondering the eternal question of life: What's the point of housework?

# The Philosophy of Housework

My dictionary describes 'philosophical' as:
'having or showing a calm attitude toward disappointments or difficulties'.

The domestic realm is a wealth of disappointments and difficulties, and for both mental and physical health, a calm attitude is the Holy Grail. So, perhaps in dealing with the undeniably futile nature of most housework, it may help to take a philosophical view and attempt a degree of acceptance. In the home, as in life, there are times when the most helpful thing to say is, 'That's just the way it is'.

Throughout the ages, many of the world's thinkers have found solace in the acceptance of certain truths, such as: life is a series of never-ending cycles; everything changes; nothing lasts forever. In my musings on the nature of domestic strife, I've come to realise that housework is a microcosm of life in general.

> There was no need to do any housework at all. After the first four years, the dirt doesn't get any worse.
>
> Quentin Crisp

Within the home, as beyond it, there are constant cycles, flows and rhythms. And the universal laws that govern our very existence apply just as much to cooking and cleaning.

Learning and accepting these philosophies will lead to finding more peace with our lot, following possibly the best advice of all time - 'go with the flow'. After all, the alternative - endless struggle against invincible forces - sounds like a lot of work.

And haven't we got enough to do?

## The Rhythm of Life

When I first took on the role of homemaker*, the aspects that I most struggled with were the repetition and monotony. I didn't mind the work, as such (well, most of it), but I was vexed by the frequency with which it needed doing.

---

*I am uncomfortable referring to myself as a housewife. Not only am I at odds with all the social implications of the title, but given my reluctance to housework, it feels fraudulent. I could be rightfully sued under the Trades Descriptions Act.

So it was with joy that I stumbled across the following passage from Roger Lanphear's book, *Wealth Consciousness*. 'Everything around us, whether from nature or man-made, uses a principle of repeating action. Without repeating action, the physical world would collapse. Rhythms are essential. Even time is a function of rhythm...All aspects of creation are involved in constant repetition...all around us as a never-ending display.'

Life, nature, our very existence is based on repetitive rhythms. Our breath, our heartbeats, seconds and minutes, days and years, the seasons, birth and death, the movement of the planets. It would seem the Grand Plan is a function of endless cycles.

Yet we don't often examine the logic of these natural laws on the larger scale. Have you ever questioned the point of spring? Or evening? Or a newborn baby? Even if we do ponder these mysteries, it is not usually on a daily basis or with begrudging misery.

Yet, a home is a vessel of lives being lived, and subject to the same natural laws of the universe. Admittedly, it is on a more mundane scale than the solar system, but the same rules apply.

So we ought not to be surprised or resentful when we are faced with the same needs, over and over. The cooking will always be followed by the washing up which will (all too swiftly) be followed by more cooking. We will wear clothes which will need washing and ironing only to become soiled again. But to fight or resent these inevitable facts is possibly the greatest waste of effort. Even if we cannot joyfully embrace the more menial rhythms of life, we will find more peace if we attempt to accept them.

Resistance truly is futile.

## Change for the better

Everything changes. Always has, always will. Few people would dispute this fact, though some will struggle with it. However, it's possible to put a positive spin on this. If there are elements of your life, your routine or your obligations that you are unhappy with, ultimately, these will change. It may or may not be in your hands to instigate the changes but it can be encouraging just to realise that any current difficulties will not last forever. People will

> The only thing constant in life is change.
>
> *François de la Rochefoucauld*

naturally move in and out of our lives. Circumstances can evolve in surprising directions. Children will grow.

Acknowledging the inevitability of change is also a good reason to start noticing and enjoying what's great about your life now. It's true that even the good stuff won't last forever, but don't be saddened by this. Instead, let this knowledge encourage you to focus on the positives in your life and truly appreciate them whilst they're around. Your life will evolve anyway, so better to have fully engaged in the best bits so you can remember them fondly, than to miss them and regret them when it's too late.

Although Joni Mitchell claimed that you don't know what you've got till it's gone - that too is subject to change.

## The Joy of Impermanence

A principle of Buddhism is that, since nothing lasts, attachment to anything is futile and can only lead to suffering. To some extent, I can relate to this. For example, let's say I spend a number of hours cleaning and tidying the house. (It does happen... occasionally.) When finished, I will stand back and admire my achievements, proud of my efforts, delighted with my beautiful home. But will it last? No, it will not. And if I get attached to it being utterly perfect, I'm going to be very unhappy. If there are people living in my home, it is inevitably going to take on that 'lived-in' look.

> Everything flows and nothing abides, everything gives way and nothing stays fixed.
>
> *Heraclitus*

So, in the pursuit of calm and serenity, it can help to accept impermanence. Enjoy things, by all means - while they last - but know that they won't last forever. When the time comes for things to fall away, an enlightened mind won't fight the inevitable. If something gets dirty or eaten or untidied, that was always going to happen, sooner or later.

Equally, as the tidiness won't last, neither will the mess. It will be dealt with, one way or another, as it always has. Such is the ebb and flow of habitation, order to mess to order to mess, ad infinitum.

We often get so wound up in the minute details of our everyday lives that we fail to see the bigger picture. Taking this broader view occasionally can help you see the pattern of existence - nothing lasts forever - and it makes perfect sense. So practice putting minor mishaps and disappointments into perspective. Don't look at a sink full of pots and decide it's a reflection of your life. It's just a sink full of pots and it will soon be behind you. (And there are far worse things you could be facing.)

Keeping this in mind will make it easier to stop fighting what was inevitable. And, with a more peaceful heart you'll see that, in the overall scheme of life, it matters not.

# Have a Scarlett O'Hara Moment

So, you've spent your time cooking or cleaning or washing or ironing etc, then you look around a few hours later and the fruits of your labours are *gone with the wind*.

Take a deep breath - it's time for a Scarlett O'Hara moment.

## Tomorrow is another day

It's true that there's an element of futility in the domestic regime - but does it do any good to agonise over it *every single time* we perform the same routine? No, it does no good, and could possibly do much harm.

So here's a little trick to help you postpone/reduce your angst: Make a decision to simply not worry about the futility of it - *at the moment*.

This takes the sting out of the problem, temporarily. Intending to worry about it another day is far easier than trying to write it off completely. You're not trying to deny your frustration (which is difficult and also unhealthy), you're just filing it for future attention.

But the real beauty of this tactic is that, often, you will forget to worry about it at all! It's a great feeling to remember that you forgot to worry about something. Especially if it turned out fine and now you don't need to bother!

> Well, I guess
> I've done murder.
> I won't think about
> that now.
> I'll think about
> that tomorrow...
>
> *Scarlett O'Hara*
>
> *(in Margaret Mitchell's Gone With The Wind)*

Even if you only manage this trick on every other attempt - you will have reduced your angst by half! So the next time you feel beaten by the utter futility of it all, take a tip from one of literature's greatest heroines. Plan to worry about it tomorrow.

# Catch the highlights

Pictures and photographs are powerful tools in obliterating feelings of pointlessness.

## Surround yourself

The photographs we take and treasure tend to be of our life's highlights. These are usually the good times; holidays, birthdays, weddings, travels, achievements, etc. Making the effort to frame these and display them all over your home can work wonders on your emotional state and overall sense of well-being. On the days when you feel your life is nothing but housework, catching a glimpse of a photograph can lift your spirits and change your mood.

> A picture is worth a thousand words.
>
> *Proverb*

Being visual, photographs work instantly. They are a fast-track connection to those happy moments, express reminders of what life really is all about. But in addition to being an effective antidote to feelings of futility, they also serve to remind you *who* you are making all this effort for and why. It's hard to dwell on 'what's the point...?' when faced with a fond memory of your loved ones.

So fill your home with images of the times you've enjoyed and the people you love. Place some in prominent positions, for regular quick fixes, but also have some in more subtle places - coming across a forgotten photograph during your domestic efforts can provoke a much-needed smile.

## Swap and change

To make the most of these effects, you'll need to move or update your photos or pictures fairly regularly. The brain quickly gets used to familiar sights and, in time, learns to ignore them. So the more often you see an image, the less impact it has. It loses its charm. Simply changing the positions of your photos will encourage you to notice them again, so swap them around as you see fit.

Also, keep updating old pictures with new ones. People, particularly children, change over time and though a little nostalgia is nice, avoid living too much in the past. Try to keep a balance of old and new.

Living in, and appreciating, the present is undoubtedly the healthiest of mental attitudes - so as wonderful new experiences occur in your life, surround yourself with the photographic evidence.

## Images of the future

You needn't limit yourself to images from the past or present. Why not put up pictures of any places you'd like to go or things you'd like to do? These can be cheering, inspiring and motivating. They can help to lift your thoughts from the drudgery of everyday chores to fun ideas of what life could have in store...beyond housework.

A common claim within success psychology is that images train the subconscious mind, which is so powerful, it can actually guide you towards whatever images it regularly receives! So, if you fancy a trip to Paris - stick a picture of the Eiffel Tower on your fridge! Theories abound about how this works, but even without scientific proof, if picturing your dreams for the future makes you feel better about your present situation, just enjoy the magic.

## Worth the dusting

Perhaps you're thinking: more photographs equals more items to dust. Technically you're right. However I believe that the benefits vastly outweigh this fact. Would you rather dust ten items miserably, or a dozen items with a smile? Whilst minimalism may be the easiest decor to keep clean, a house should feel like a home, not just an efficient shell. It is the personal items that make your home unique. In fact - they are what make it *home*.

# Is joy futile?

## The joy of giving

Although we humans have a strong self-serving instinct, there can be times when we wouldn't bother to do something for ourselves, but the impulse to care for another means we'd willingly do it for them.

For example, some days I'd quite happily forgo a home-cooked dinner in favour of something quick and easy. However, I find dishing up a sumptuous meal to my family quite satisfying, so doing it for them can be more of a motivation.

But once the meal is over, was it a futile exercise? The food is gone and the tribe will be hungry again in a matter of hours, so what was the point?

Well, there may be no tangible evidence of my efforts, but caring for others and enjoying myself are also valid results of my time. So, not only are my family well-fed (result), they feel cared for (result) and I spent a happy hour doing something I enjoy (result!).

It's possible, though, that the frequency and repetition of having to provide this service dilutes/obliterates any inherent joy. But if it falls to you to fulfill these tasks, you may as well look for ways to enjoy them. One way to do this is to focus on each event in isolation, rather than remembering all the times past it had to be done. Once you get past the psychological baggage, you may be surprised how many occasions you find enjoyment in your schedule. (No, honestly!)

Just because a job is supposedly futile, that doesn't mean it can't be satisfying - *if you open yourself up this possibility*. Performing a service for others has a value in and of itself - regardless of the end result. There is, or at least, there can be enjoyment in giving or caring or providing a service. It is rewarding, i.e., you get a reward. That sounds like a result to me.

## Varying degrees of loathing

Do you absolutely detest every single chore? Aren't there some that you don't actually mind too much, or even, dare I say it ...enjoy? If you answer *no*, feel free to skip this bit, but do think carefully first.

To give you a personal example - I'm the first to admit that I am as far from naturally domestic as it is possible to be, but even I find a strange pleasure in cleaning windows. Maybe it's the transformation from grubby panes of shame to a sparkling, diamond shine to be proud of. Or perhaps it's my homemade squirty-bottle concoction of vinegar and water, or the satisfying streak-free buffing with a paper towel.

Whatever the reason, I find it an effective, efficient and relatively easy route to feeling like a competent homemaker (at least, until a dust bunny scuttles past me...). However, this admission doesn't mean that I live to clean windows. I don't. But when even I have to admit that they need doing, I console myself with the thought that it's not my least favourite job.

So ponder your routine and try to rediscover any potential areas of enjoyment. It may be that, at least in some cases, you don't begrudge the work, as such; it's just your 'issues' that take the shine off any joy.

Resenting every job is exhausting, so if you must focus on how much you loathe them, at least loathe them by degrees.

## Treading water

OK, so logic suggests that there's no point doing housework. It will only be undone and/or need doing again. However, life is not merely about efficiencies. Do you want to exist logically or live happily? There is one major reason to bother with seemingly futile maintenance: the alternative. Avoiding squalor, illness, chaos, stress and misery are all worthwhile reasons for an element of effort.

If you called a halt on housework, the dust, mess and grime will carry on regardless. So you would, eventually, be swallowed up by deterioration and neglect. To maintain ourselves, our families and our homes may not be seen as a progression, as such, but it is certainly an achievement. Our lives are better for the effort - so technically, that's an improvement of sorts.

> What is important in life is life, and not the result of life.
>
> *Johann Wolfgang von Goethe*

In keeping on top of the domestic schedule, we may not be advancing, but at least we're not being dragged down either. Think of it as treading water; it might not get you anywhere, but if you stop - you're sunk!

## Pleasure-seeker

Beyond basic requirements for health and sanity, the sole point of doing some jobs is that you feel better when they're done - logic or not.

Let's just examine that... *you feel better.* So if it makes you feel better, it's absolutely worthwhile! What is life about, if not to feel good? If you've discovered a technique to doing that - why would you not do it?

You may not particularly enjoy the effort but focus on how much you enjoy the result. Most things worth having come with a price of some sort - and usually the sweeter for it. So if getting certain jobs done makes you feel better than if you left them - what are you waiting for?

> It takes patience to appreciate domestic bliss; volatile spirits prefer unhappiness.
>
> *George Santayana*

Of course, you get to decide which prices you're willing to pay - it's a personal thing. For example, I could go on at length on the futility of the washing-up (and quite often do...) but there is no denying the satisfaction I feel when my kitchen is spotless, compared to the utter desolation of it being a mess.

So select the results that make you smile. Decide once and for all that the outcome is worth the effort, then there's no need to question the futility *every time you do them.* This will release all that mental angst, wondering if you're wasting your life. Then you can just get on with those tasks, knowing that they're worth doing, simply because they are worthwhile *for you.*

# The power of habits

One way to avoid dwelling on the depressing futility of certain tasks is to learn how to do them without thinking.

Getting some of your workload done *on autopilot*, i.e., without your conscious awareness or focus, will massively reduce those feelings of pointlessness. So, if you have unavoidable chores where the frequency and regularity is driving you mind - it's time to harness the awesome power of your unconscious mind.

## Brain-training

Re-occurring jobs come to feel pointless because you devote your mental energy to them on a regular basis. But what if you could train your brain to perform those annoying tasks - without you noticing? This may sound a bit extreme, but think about it: you do it already.

Do you ponder the futility of taking a breath in, followed by a breath out, over and over and over, day after day? No, you just do it without thinking. Your subconscious mind is in charge and just gets on with it without bothering you for your attention. No doubt you can think of other things you do without thinking (as absurd as this may sound). In fact, you may have some practices that are so strongly entrenched that you actually can't help doing them. I have a friend who folds everything in sight. She doesn't even realise she's doing it but if you asked her to stop - she couldn't!

So how can this help us? One word: habits. We can (if we choose) control our habits, both good and bad. They are just wiring patterns in our brains which get stronger by doing something over and over again, until they become automatic. But the brain can be reprogrammed, so bad habits can be broken and good habits can be created.

Time for a practical example. Let's say your most irksome task is cleaning the loo. Why not *get into the habit* of giving it a quick wipe/ brush every time you 'perform your daily ablutions'? Now this might sound too much like hard work to begin with. (I'm with you on that score.) But I know many women who swear by this practice and have been doing it for so long that it is automatic. They don't wonder if they can be bothered, *they don't think about it at all* - auto-pilot kicks in and, magically, it's done!

This practice has the triple-bonus of a) eliminating the mental misery of knowing it needs doing, b) the job becomes the work of moments when done daily and c) the not-to-be-underestimated satisfaction of knowing that your toilet is always clean.

That enviable feeling of being effortlessly on top of your workload is completely within your grasp - simply by setting new habit patterns! Theories vary about how long it takes to create or break a habit, although the general consensus is somewhere between 3 and 4 weeks, but my advice is just keep doing it until you no longer notice that you're doing it.

Accept that it may feel frustratingly difficult - at first. This is just your resistance that you have allowed to get a foothold - but you can break this down. Decide if you're committed (review the bonuses above), then keep at it. You will break the habit of trying to avoid the job and in its place will be a much more supportive and efficient one.

The mind is an amazingly powerful tool, yet vastly underused; experts believe we only use a fraction of its potential. So start using this free, natural resource to your advantage! You are the controller - you just need to 'put your mind to it'. Unless you're fond of dwelling on how unhappy your jobs make you, why not hand over a bit of your domestic angst to your subconscious mind?

Don't you dream of an assistant to take some of your workload off your hands? Well, it is, quite literally, in your head.

# Time-wasting

What's your definition of a waste of time?

## Get comfortable with non-achieving

Our culture is fast-paced and highly pressured. It's normal to try and cram as many activities as possible into every waking moment. Multitasking and high achieving are seen as the ultimate use of our time.

In this light, it's difficult to see housework as an effective endeavour. In terms of tangible and lasting evidence of achievement, menial chores about the home don't score very highly.

However, the recent trend in downshifting would suggest that this constant craving for attainment is not the route to a happy life. People are increasingly finding that this never-ending frenzy of activity is actually quite unfulfilling or not their preferred way to live. Often this realisation is followed by radical life changes, just to get a little more time out, a little more *life*. Downshifters want to achieve less and live more. They often find a renewed joy and appreciation for life's simpler activities such as… wait for it... cooking, gardening, and caring for the home!

But it is not necessary (and certainly not desirable) to reach the point of burn-out before you stop chasing things that won't bring you happiness. If you start to view success in terms of health, happiness and quality of life, you can let go of the constant pressure to achieve.

This attitude is filtering through into society where the achievement-focused mania of previous decades is making room for an appreciation of enjoying the moment. Less getting and having, more doing and being. Success is beginning to be measured, not solely in terms of salary or house size, but by amount of quality time with family, opportunities to pursue hobbies, travel, relaxation, exciting experiences, the extent of health and stress-free living.

This time spent on experiencing pleasure as opposed to obtaining results is not time wasted - *it is life lived!*

> Enjoy the little things, for one day you may look back and realise they were the big things.
>
> *Robert Brault*

So, if there is merit in activities that achieve nothing other than enjoyment, pleasure, love and health - doesn't housework fall into this category? There are few more simple, basic, stress-free, and ultimately rewarding activities than tending to your environment (that is, if you have a positive mental attitude towards it). Even if housework is not your favourite pastime, spending time on your home is an investment in the experience you have there, i.e., making it enjoyable, loving, supportive and healthy. It's an investment in the quality of not just your home life, but your whole life.

Satisfaction and enjoyment are the results of housework, if not during, then at least afterwards. Yet, if you still feel the need to question the point of doing things purely for pleasure, go beyond caring for your home and family. What about watching TV - what's the point of that? Or reading, gardening, playing, relaxing, etc... If you spend a couple of hours at the cinema - what does that achieve? Spending time with someone you love may have no physical result but is it a waste of time? How often do you worry about the efficiency of the time you spend sleeping or bathing or eating? Is it futile to do these things? After all, they will only need doing again.

If you happily devote your time to other leisure or health-giving activities which produce either immediate enjoyment or long term benefits - why struggle with the idea of housework?

Letting go of the need to achieve things - *all the time* - can liberate you to find the joy in your present experience, regardless of the outcome. And focussing on the job in hand, rather than your resentment of it, will be an infinitely more pleasant experience.

So why not give yourself a break from constantly judging your tasks on their overall results, or focusing on what else you could be doing? Then, as you get comfortable with just being in the moment, the non-achieving aspect of housework will bother you so much less.

## Results a go go

Alternatively... If you are a dyed-in-the-wool high achiever and cannot come to terms with a lack of results, it may help you to view housework as the ultimate multi-tasking activity. With a closer examination of the work you do within the home, you'll discover that you are actually producing results all over the place!

**Life improver.** Whether you are an advocate of feng shui or not, housework (or a lack thereof) undoubtedly affects the *feel* of a room or home, which in turn affects the inhabitants. So in tending to your home, you're not merely cleaning and tidying, you are impacting the unseen energy patterns in the lives of those you live with. You may never know the direct results of your labours, but if there are invisible forces at work, wouldn't you prefer to unleash the positive ones?

**Femme fitale.** Housework is a valid form of exercise which, as you know, is good for you. It can be as vigorous or as gentle as you like. It is low impact and unlikely to inflict injuries. Thus you are houseworking your way to a healthier you. This is a double whammy result - cleaner home and thinner thighs!

**Career girl.** Money experts agree that whatever invisible hands direct success our way, they do so much more effectively in tidy and organised situations. I used to think it coincidental that more work flowed my way after a good office tidy-up but it has happened to me so frequently and predictably that I know there's something in it.

Investing time and energy in the upkeep of your home is not a polar opposite of your career - it can actually enhance it. I'll repeat that, in case you missed the enormity of that one statement. *Investing time and energy in the upkeep of your home is not a polar opposite of your career - it can actually enhance it.*

**Bright spark.** Rhythmical, repetitive actions, especially if carried out on auto-pilot, lull your brain into a meditative state. This alpha rhythm is highly conducive to creativity - when you are most likely to be struck by inspired thought, right-brain insights, brilliant ideas and intuitive prompts. Have you ever found yourself in the middle of your chores and the solution to a recent quandary 'mysteriously' popped into your head? When your brain is in housework mode, it quietly deals with complex problems without you even noticing. So, you're not just vacuuming - you're channeling your genius!

## Doing your bit

Do you ever see those charity ads on TV or in the mail and feel a pang of guilt that you really could do more to contribute to the world?

Well, the next time you feel that way, don't be so hard on yourself - just think of all the thankless effort you put into your home and family! If you do the amount of housework attributed to the average woman then you're already making a substantial contribution.

So housework is not completely pointless - it's an act of charity! Doing voluntary work, for the benefit of others without recognition or financial reward, counts just as much within your own four walls as it does within the community or further afield.

We often find it easier to give unconditionally to total strangers than to our loved ones. But if we can learn to be more benevolent to our family - carrying out the work in a spirit of charity - it will automatically feel more worthwhile, and indeed worthy. Of course, you can always do good works outside your home, as well, but that is a personal decision. Just know that taking care of a home and/or family is an act of giving, and doing this goes some way towards doing your bit - for which you should be proud.

> If you haven't any charity in your heart, you have the worst kind of heart trouble.
>
> *Bob Hope*

So try to stop keeping score or expecting a return on your efforts, which all too often leads to disappointment and frustration. If you are going to do the work anyway, doing it with a willing and generous heart turns it into a meaningful act of giving. Charity can be a donation of time, as well as money. And when that charity begins at home - it's time well spent.

## Moment by moment

Memory plays a significant role in creating a sense of futility. You may feel that you're just wasting your time in a certain task purely because you have done it so many times already. So try judging each occasion on its own merits, without all the baggage from the past. Instead of bemoaning, *I need to clean the kitchen, just like I have done every day since blah blah blah...* (and the depressing spiral of misery *that* provokes) just rephrase it calmly in your mind - *I need to clean the kitchen today.*

It doesn't help in any way to dwell miserably on how many times you've done it in the past. There's nothing you can do about that now. Deal with the present, the only place you have any control. Also, don't contemplate how many times you may have to do it in the future. Who knows what's around the corner?

So face each day afresh. Put yesterday behind you and worry about tomorrow when it arrives. Your sense of futility will be radically diminished as you just deal with one day at a time.

## Short-term effort, long-term results

Do you dwell on the futility of brushing your teeth? Most likely you just get on with it because the consequences of not brushing aren't very appealing (bad breath, inflamed gums, rotting, black or missing teeth... need I go on?)

Oral hygiene (like much domestic work) is a monotonous, regular activity with no immediately visible results - yet we don't question whether it's worth doing. So why do we dwell on the pointlessness of housework? The consequences of skipping that are equally grim.

So, instead of wondering whether it is a good use of your time, perhaps consider what will happen if you 'save' time by not doing housework...

**Well, well, well.** Housework may be repetitive but it is this aspect which prevents the build-up or infestation of germs and microbial undesirables. These little beasties never tire of their mission to infiltrate our homes and bodies. The only effective defence is constant guard and frequent eradication. If we drop this effort, we are liable to pay with our health and well-being. Safeguarding your health is a worthwhile effort, both in the long- and short-term, because preventing illness is actually less time-consuming (and unpleasant) than being ill.

**Coming up roses.** Pooh! Bad smells! Foul odours within the home are actually quite helpful barometers that something requires attention - but they are not very popular! Aside from their unpleasantness, there is a social stigma - nobody wants to think that others regard their house as smelly. So if you don't wish your home to be known as Pooh Corner, constant vigilance and odour management will be required.

**Organize and conquer.** You waste infinitely more time falling over or searching for things if you live in a mess, than is required to tidy or organize your stuff in the first place. The problem here is trying to keep the long-term view. Yes, it is easier - in the short-term - to just dump stuff or leave it out and it can be tempting to do so. But try to remember that there will be a time-cost for this approach.

Jobs invariably take longer to do when left. Also, you are less efficient in the midst of chaos than in an organized environment when everything is in its place. Being disorganized or untidy is not only time-consuming but stressful. Think of lost keys when running late - now does that small, short-term effort seem so difficult by comparison?

**Heart and home.** How do you react emotionally when your home is in a sorry state? Your home affects your mood, and given the time you spend there, it plays an enormous part in your overall emotional state and consequently, every aspect of your life. This fact alone makes the nurturing of it immensely worthwhile. You take the effects of your home with you when you leave it. It is your base, the foundation for the rest of your life. Looking after your personal space provides a place that supports you and prepares you for dealing with the world beyond your door. It's your sanctuary. The time investment in its care and upkeep will reap rewards in every area of your life.

**Mess vs success.** Even if you dodge serious illness from poor hygiene, living in chaos and grubbiness is not particularly pleasant, neither is it conducive to success and vitality. The hallmarks of most successful people are organisation, orderliness and immaculate presentation of their person and invariably their home (even if much of this work is delegated...) So why not appeal to your aspirational side? Tidy your way to success! Have you ever noticed how much happier and more positive you feel after a good sort-out or a thorough clean? Unleashing this vibrant, positive energy into your home and your life can transform your circumstances. Unless your life is already perfect, why not give it a go? Taking the time to make the place clean and tidy can truly invite the good stuff in.

Although it is possible to enjoy housework (no, really!), even if you don't, there is much value in the long-term benefits. All that invisible work has invisible rewards - physically, financially, emotionally, mentally, even spiritually. It may be hard to imagine or appreciate this in the midst of constant effort but these benefits are substantial. They are good and valid reasons to 'waste your time' on housework.

Your domestic efforts contribute to the smooth running and enjoyment of your life and those you live with. By keeping your home well, you're not merely providing a pleasant environment in which to live - you are sowing the seeds for your future health, wealth and happiness.

Can you think of a better use of your time?

Section 4:

# no energy

Fight fatigue?

I don't have the energy.

# If only I had more energy...

Has your get-up-and-go got up and gone?

In the battle against housework, you need to be well armed on the energy front. If your energy levels are low, you will be toast. Housework is demanding and only the strong have a hope of surviving. But if you currently feel you're neither strong nor surviving, fear not! There is much you can do to improve matters. And best of all, for some of the following suggestions, you won't need to lift a finger.

All you will need, to begin with, is an intention to do something positive about your energy levels. This first and vital step will see you well along the road to improvements. So relax, take a deep breath (no, really do - it's a great energiser), and get ready for the new, bouncy, bubbly, vibrant and dynamic you!

## Plugging the leaks

The ideas in this section deal mainly with boosting your energy. However, we're all *naturally energetic*, so if you're missing out on your innate resources of vitality - something must be sapping them. Taking steps to increase your energy levels is great but if your energy is still being drained by negative forces, you will make slow progress, if any at all. This is why an effective first step on the road to more energy is to plug any unnecessary leaks.

Attitudes toward housework can be one such leak. Although housework is basically physical labour, if you have 'issues' with the work itself, it may be robbing you of considerable mental or emotional energy as well. Stress is an insidious energy-sapper, so if your domestic role frequently stresses you out, it's little wonder you lack the energy to cope.

In her book *Fight Fatigue*, Mary Ann Bauman suggests that energy problems arise not so much from what work you have to do, *but from how you feel about it*. If you have any emotional or mental resistance, the task will drain you.

Perhaps you can relate to this if you've ever felt resistance to housework (and who hasn't?). Luckily, this problem can be fixed relatively simply - by a shift in attitude. Finding a new insight or more positive mindset could free up extra energy before you even start. (Giving you more chance of actually getting started.)

So it can be helpful, then, to make a point of unearthing your domestic demons. The first step is to try and identify them. Are there particular chores that make you just want to go back to bed? Try to discover exactly what it is that causes this reaction. Sometimes, this step alone will shed some light on the problem, enabling you to see a solution. Another tactic is to discuss it with a friend, parent, spouse, even your child (children often have a refreshing take on matters.) Alternatively, do a quick search on the internet to see if anyone else suffers from the same issue and what they did to cope.

Nature abhors
a vacuum.
And so do I.

*Anne Gibbons*

Hopefully the contents of this book will short-cut your search for new perspectives and enlightening insights. In fact, the whole concept was born of my analysis as to why housework throws up so many psychological issues. So, if you haven't already done so, you may want to check out the other sections that deal specifically with negative attitudes towards housework.

However you choose to plug the leaks, this step is essential if you want to permanently increase your energy levels to enable you to cope more easily with your home and family. This alone will automatically release more of your natural vitality.

Once you have dealt with drains on your mental energy, it's time to look at ways of increasing your levels of physical energy. And for that, all you need to do is take your pick from the pages ahead. Some of the ideas require nothing more than a slight adjustment in your habits. Many of the suggestions are easy and fun, and some are positively indulgent! Of course, there are ideas which call for some effort on your part, but taking responsibility and action is empowering. The simple decision to take back the reins of your life is, in itself, is a fantastic energiser.

## The Domino Effect

Before we embark on the solutions, however, it can be useful to consider why energy problems have arisen in the first place - if only to prevent ourselves sliding back into energy-sapping ways in the future.

Our energy levels are a result of many factors. We humans are complicated. We're an intricate function of many processes and elements - and many of these are related. Although we recognise different types of energy, e.g., physical, mental, emotional, etc... they are all interlinked. If you affect one, you affect the others. So a deficiency in one area can manifest as a problem elsewhere. For example, when you are emotionally wrung out, you lack physical vitality and mental alertness.

Sluggish physical energy, then, may actually be a result of a mental or emotional issue. Although diet and exercise undoubtedly play a huge role in your physical energy levels, any good works can be compromised if you have a problem that is sapping you psychologically or emotionally.

Happily though, this connection works both ways. When you improve one aspect of your well-being, there are positive repercussions across the board! This is the philosophy behind holistic healthcare, such as the branch of Eastern medicine known as Ayurveda. For a practical example of this domino effect, consider how physical exercise can increase mental clarity, or soothe a heartache.

Although it can certainly be helpful to investigate what's causing your depleted energy, it's not necessary to know whether your problems are physical, emotional or mental, since an improvement in any area will lead to benefits overall. (Besides, the suggestions that follow will cover all three areas, some simultaneously.) In this way, as you take any steps towards boosting your energy, you will embark on an upward spiral to ultimately regain your natural sparkle.

So feel free to choose whichever suggestions take your fancy (your instinct knows what you need). Or better still, try them all - and just watch your energy levels soar!

Please note, though: the following ideas are solutions to general malaise. If you are suffering from a serious, debilitating fatigue, this could be a symptom of something more serious than Housework Blues and may require medical or professional treatment. Equally, any exercise or dietary suggestions are given on the understanding that, if necessary, you first consult your doctor.

That said, there is little (if anything) that follows that can do any harm - and will most likely do much good. So if you're ready, willing and able - come on, jump in! The energy's lovely...

# Looking after No.1

Women are instinctive nurturers and carers. Historically, we are the caretakers of the species. Even in recent times, women who work full-time still tend to be the ones who make a house a home, administer TLC and know/care how each family member likes their breakfast. Regardless of who has the earning power, it's usually the Lady of the House who manages the everyday comings and goings. She-Who-Knows-Where-The-Clean-Socks-Are (or aren't, perhaps).

Now, whether we like this idea or not, it's in our genes (though admittedly stronger in some women than others...) In any home, the family-support mechanism tends to stem from the resident female.

Consequently, we often find ourselves at the beck and call of others. In demand. Needed. This is obviously important in the raising of infants, but when and where do we draw the line? At what point should we say, *What about my needs? Where do they rank?* A common female tendency is to put our own needs on hold. The trouble is, they often get pushed so far down the list that they get neglected or forgotten completely.

But this selflessness could be doing a disservice to both ourselves and those who rely on us. Firstly, self-interest is human nature. In stifling our wants and needs, we're inhibiting a basic human urge. Ultimately, suppressing what we want from life is a recipe for disaster. We each have personal desires and goals - to bury these will inevitably lead to resentment. Resentment is not only unhealthy, it can only be tolerated for so long. Sooner or later, it will rear its head - usually with unpleasant results.

> Self-preservation,
> nature's first great law,
> all the creatures,
> except man, doth awe.
>
> *Andrew Marvell*

Even Buddhism, which is renowned for its charitable philosophies, concedes that we should have moderation in all. Although we've been taught to consider others - and compassion, empathy and kindness undoubtedly play a part in a good life - it ought not to be at the total exclusion of our own needs. By all means, take care of those you love. If it makes you happy to do things for people, go ahead. Just make sure you're not always bottom of the list.

Secondly, as Mother Nature, success gurus, even air-hostesses all know - self-preservation is paramount. It's the first law of nature. Your first responsibility is keeping yourself alive - you cannot help anybody else, if you don't achieve this. To do justice to yourself, others and society as a whole, you need to meet your own basic needs first.

But even beyond basic survival, you'll be so much better placed to take care of your home and family if you're fit and well, full of energy and joy. The pleasure you get from regularly meeting your own needs will make you much more willing to give of yourself. In this way, being selfish is a selfless act!

This self-maintenance will take work, though, or at least time and effort. So you may need to make a commitment, to dedicate some space in your life for your self-care. If you're not used to prioritising what *you* want, you might feel uneasy, at first, but it's worth persevering. There will almost certainly be a time cost and you may feel that you're denying your family some of their needs, but this reasoning is short-term. If you *don't* do these vital, nurturing things (for yourself), there will come a time when you aren't in a position to help your family - or you may lack the inclination to do so. Neither scenario is in anyone's best interests.

Eating well, getting enough sleep, staying healthy, finding calm, doing activities that bring you joy - all these things involve a commitment to you but it is one that will reap benefits for everybody. So make *you* a priority. It's not a selfish endeavour - you're actually investing in your long-term ability to help and serve others. Happily.

Plus, one of the many benefits of proper self-care is energy, so it's a win-win situation. By prioritising your me-time, you're far more likely to have the energy to provide care and support for the ones you love. In looking after No.1, you are ensuring you'll have the energy to be there for those who need you.

## But I don't have time...

If your main concern is taking care of a home and family, you'll fare so much better if you are in optimum health. All the other skills required to run a home are worthless without the health to administer them. For this reason alone, health should be top of the list of things you make time for.

Admittedly, in our busy modern lives, it can be easy to neglect our physical and mental well-being, at least until something goes wrong. But prevention is always preferable to cure, so timetable your health needs, if nothing else. *Make time for them.* And this includes your mental well-being, too. If you need regular rest and relaxation to feel good, schedule it in! It's not indulgent. R&R is a basic human need - not a luxury. If you deny yourself this, I guarantee those around you will feel it.

> If you nurture your mind, body, and spirit, your time will expand.
>
> *Brian Koslow*

So prioritise your wellness. If you still need persuading to meet your own needs - see it as an act of giving. Making time to look after yourself will result in a more fulfilled and healthful version of you, which is truly a gift to those around you - and the world beyond.

## Energy and self-esteem

Your self-esteem and your energy levels are closely related. You seldom find people with low self-esteem to be full of vivacious energy. So in our bid to boost your energy - check in with your self-esteem.

How do you value yourself? Sometimes (though not always) a desire to run around after everybody else is linked to low self-worth - as if everybody else's needs are more important than yours. If this is the case, by valuing yourself more (i.e., prioritising your self-care), you will benefit doubly from increased energy. As you begin to take better care of yourself, you will feel more energetic. But a side effect will be improved self-esteem and as this increases - your energy will too!

You can also expect another happy side effect: When we acknowledge our own worth, others will do the same. When you respect and honour yourself, others respond with renewed respect. So, if you feel unappreciated and undervalued, start appreciating and valuing *yourself!* Other people are often a mirror of how we view ourselves, so you have to value yourself first, before you can expect others to. Plus, a sense of being unappreciated is a negative emotion. Negativity drains your natural vibrancy and sparkle, so by releasing this, you get yet another boost to your energy levels.

Meeting your own needs and desires is a sure way of recognising your own worth, and bringing about the benefits of improved self-esteem. Plus it's fun! Indeed, some would argue that's why we are here - to have a joyful and fulfilling experience!

So, add 'Me' to your list of things that matter. Your self-esteem and generosity will increase, your energy levels will rise and your family will value and appreciate this new, vivacious you.

All this just by looking after No.1. Not the most unpleasant sacrifice you could make...

## Now for the fun bit...

Now that we've established that it's an essential, worthy and selfless act to take care of yourself, we can explore the joy in what that entails.

How would you like to book yourself a massage? A manicure? An exercise class? A shopping trip? A holiday all by yourself? How would you like to curl up with a book? Or watch a film? Or go out dancing? Do it! Do them all! Being happy and fulfilled is good for you. It keeps you fit and well and generous of spirit - it can even keep you young!

Do more of what you love to do, whatever that may be. You'll be amazed at how the time and resources miraculously become available once you decide that it's the right thing to do. Men know it! Generally speaking, they don't have this tendency to suppress their own needs. Of course, many men are loving and giving to

> Remember the entrance door to the sanctuary is inside you.
>
> *Rumi*

their families - but on the whole, they're pretty good at eking out their fair share of fun. And it's only right. Regardless of your responsibilities and commitments, *you also matter.* As much as anybody else.

So keep the self-sacrificing in check and get down to some serious 'me-time'.

You really are worth it.

# Ditch the Sappers

Do you ever suffer from:

- Indecision?
- Procrastination?
- Stress?
- Exhaustion?

In today's busy world, it's a rare person who escapes all of the above. And within the home, the workload can be made even more challenging by these energy-drainers. Wondering when (or if) to do certain tasks robs you of mental energy. The stress of drowning in domestic work can be emotionally draining. And the exhaustion that comes from constantly chasing your tail can leave you physically wiped out.

Time to ditch these sappers!

The good news is that there are simple measures you can take, small habits you can adopt to offset these drains on your natural resources. These ideas are simple to understand and easy to implement, yet they will reap vast energy dividends. But here's the real magic: although your renewed vitality will mean you're more able to cope with the housework, these techniques take care of the bulk of the chores - so you can use all that extra energy for something else!

So, if the idea of more energy and less work appeals to you - get comfy and read on. We're going to plug some leaks...

## Routine therapy

Routine has a bad press. There's a sense of the mundane and predictable, unexciting even, about fixed procedures. And if excitement is what you crave, I will concede that routine systems are probably not for you. However, if what you crave is more order, less chaos and the feeling that you are in control of your home and/or your life, then routine just might be the tool for the job.

Traditionally, routine played a starring role in domestic management. The stately homes of old would have a strict timetable; laundry day, baking day, etc - and with good reason. Without this regime in place, the sheer volume of chores would have resulted in chaos. Admittedly those homes were on a grander scale than the average family residence, but the same principle applies. When there is much work to be done on an ongoing basis - you need a system.

Adopting a routine can be an effective and efficient way of getting things done. But best of all, it removes a significant amount of worry - worrying when, how or if you'll cope with it all. A sense of being overwhelmed will wreak havoc with your energy supplies. By simply scheduling your jobs into your timetable, you can relax, knowing they will be dealt with. So, no more fretting over that mountain of washing - it will be tackled on Monday. No stressing about when you'll get to the supermarket - that's a Wednesday evening task. And so on...

Though your instinct may be to kick against this much control over your life, it's worth trying to get past this resistance. If you succeed, you'll actually find that routines can be incredibly liberating. Routine will make the same amount of work appear easier, simply because you've removed all that mental angst surrounding it.

> The secret of your future is hidden in your daily routine.
>
> *Mike Murdock*

Of course, it may be difficult at first, but like any new habit, if you persevere it will soon become second nature. Then once you have a system in place that works for you, feel free to shake it up a little, if necessary. It's your life, you're in control, you get to decide the balance of order and spontaneity. Exploit the benefits of a routine but alter the detail, if that's what suits.

The idea is to use routine to your advantage. You cannot complete all your chores in one day. In fact, I hate to break it to you, but housework is ongoing - you're never going to be finished! But there is a great deal of peace in knowing that it's all in hand. It's comforting to know that your commitments have a place in your routine and you'll get to them at the appropriate time.

So give routine a try and then, when you're serene and on top of your game, I bet you'll wonder how you ever managed without it.

## Make it a policy

In many ways, managing a home is like running a business. Many of the same principles apply: efficiency, time-management, prioritising, etc. These techniques, used so successfully in the corporate realm, can also be applied within the home to improve our 'domestic business'.

One such technique is the practice of policy making. Companies large and small, even governments, recognise the importance of some ground rules. Firm policies help to resolves dilemmas or deliberation. With guidelines in place, it becomes much easier to choose the option which supports your ultimate goal.

For example, the only time I can do any 'proper work' (i.e., the stuff I get paid for) is when my youngest child is at nursery. So I have adopted a policy of no housework during his nursery sessions. Some days, when the kitchen is a mess, or the laundry is piling up, I'm tempted to 'just do this' or 'just sort that'. But in my experience this is always a mistake. I'll get sucked into all the other jobs that just need a bit of attention and before I know it, it's pick-up time and I haven't even sat down at my desk.

However, when I force myself to ignore the housework, knowing that this is in line with my previously-agreed policy, I get my work done. I determine what's necessary to achieve my goal (some work). I make some decisions about how that could happen, i.e., I set my policy, then I stick to it. (Though I have to admit, some days neglecting the housework isn't too much of a struggle...)

> Indecision is the graveyard of good intentions
>
> *Unknown*

But how will this help your energy levels? Well, indecision saps your mental energy. Having policies eliminates the deliberation. You dispense with the agonising over whether to do it now or later, what should you do first, etc. When you set a policy, you are deciding, in advance, what you will do and when. So when you're faced with uncertainty, you check in with your guidelines to know exactly what to do. This removes the energy-sapping dilemmas and the sense that there's so much to do that you don't know where to start.

On page 30, I mention the 3 Sees Rule. This is another example of using a pre-determined agreement to know how to handle situations as they come up. Although I personally find this one particularly effective, I appreciate we react differently. Decide for yourself the best route for you. However, the critical thing here is that you *decide*. Give it some thought beforehand. Figure out the way that will work for you, then stick to your plans. Set your policies, once and for all. Then you won't need to stress over each occasion. You'll easily know the right thing to do.

In the business world, the managers who become most successful are decisive. They may give thoughtful consideration when it's necessary but for the minor quandaries, they know exactly what to do. This is because they have their goals and rules firmly in mind and develop the policies that support them. Then it's easy to see which option will serve their larger aims.

In his insightful book, *The Success Principles*, Jack Canfield has a section entitled '99% is a bitch, 100% is a breeze'. Here he explains how setting your commitments and plans, once and for all, and deciding to stick to them, is actually easier than being half-hearted about it. In his words, 'It makes life easier and simpler. It frees up tons of energy that would otherwise have been spent internally debating the topic over and over.'

In this way, the energy you save wondering about it can be used to do the task in hand. This technique will set you firmly on the path toward your ultimate goals, whether that is to have a comforting home or more energy, or both.

Here's an example. Let's say your goal is to always have a spotless kitchen. In your own home, you'll know what level of commitment that requires. Knowing this, you can either choose to make that commitment, or not. If you decide to commit, you'll then need to implement strategies to achieve it. One such policy may be to wipe up spills and crumbs whenever you see them. Then, the next time you're wondering whether to clean up that spill, if you are committed to your larger goal (spotless kitchen) you don't need to wrestle with the decision. You know what you need to do and, if you're serious about what you say you want, you will just do it.

Admittedly this requires discipline, but as the late inspirational speaker Jim Rohn used to say, 'We suffer either the pain of discipline or the pain of regret. Discipline weighs ounces and regret weighs tons.'

So consider your intentions for your home, your lifestyle and your domestic responsibilities. Take time to prioritise what matters to you and devise a route to achieving it. This effort will be rewarded tenfold when you no longer waste time wondering whether to do it now or later. Or even, at all.

## Stress less

Ever get stressed? How do you feel about that? Some people love it - they thrive on the adrenaline. (Though this is ill-fated, as the body will require ever-increasing levels of stress, resulting in burn-out.) Most people, though, would like to reduce the amount of stress in their lives. This is because being over-stressed is not particularly enjoyable and the after-effects aren't great either. These include irritability, tension, headaches, lack of concentration, short-term memory loss, sadness, even fever. Oh, and stress literally eats energy.

So, why do we get stressed? Stress occurs when we're under some sort of pressure (either real or imagined). When there's a real threat of danger, stress can be helpful in initiating the fight or flight instinct. This helps us to survive. What's less helpful is the constant and destructive stress of many modern lifestyles. It seems our whole lives have become a case of too much to do in too little time. But, if we stop to consider all this, it begs the question - what's the rush?

Out there - in the world beyond our home - there may be external pressures to rush about like crazy. Deadlines and appointments may be beyond our immediate control. On home territory, though, we are in charge. We get to decide which jobs get done and when. Alright, mealtimes have a certain immovable rigidity - people tend to want feeding at regular intervals. But for most of the domestic workload, we get to call the shots.

> For fast-acting relief,
> try slowing down.
>
> *Lily Tomlin*

If we choose to, we can adopt a slower, less frenzied pace. There may be a cost - getting less done (though this is arguable) - but the rewards are significant. Firstly, you'll have a much more pleasant experience in taking care of your home. Secondly, you'll feel less drained and more fulfilled afterwards. Thirdly, you'll gain health benefits through stressing less and practicing more relaxed, contemplative methods. And finally, you will be so much more efficient when not in a rush. In fact, the combination of all these virtues results in you being more effective, energetic and capable - meaning you could actually get *more* done. So why not ditch the voluntary dashing about which is not only bad for your health - it's actually counter-productive.

Aside from our self-imposed pressures, another source of stress is racing against the clock. This occurs when everything needs doing at once, or it's all been left until the last minute. Although very common and completely normal, it's neither fun nor healthy.

But there is another way!

In exchange for a little prep work, life can run much more smoothly. How would you like to see all of your commitments beautifully coordinated and competently achieved? Not only is this possible, it's not particularly difficult. All it requires is a soupçon of discipline and a sprinkle of good habits...

> I try to take one day at a time, but sometimes several days attack me at once.
>
> Jennifer Yane

Stress occurs when we're up against it, when we're at a disadvantage in an important situation. But there are steps we can take - *in advance* - to improve our odds of coping. We can give ourselves an advantage just by being prepared. Success in any walk of life comes from adequate planning. As they say, if you fail to plan - plan to fail! Planning ahead, in a relaxed way, without the element of panic, requires very little energy. (And it's a satisfying feeling, to know you're ahead of the game.) Yet the results from this small effort can make an enormous difference to the quality of your life.

By adopting preemptive practices (e.g., routines, policies and planning), you will be more organised - almost effortlessly. If you anticipate what needs to be done - and take steps to be prepared, or even get a head start - those regular stressful situations will 'mysteriously' decrease. Though life will always throw up unforeseen challenges, when you're in control of the everyday stuff, you're less likely to be thrown off course.

So if you want to reduce your stress and increase your energy - be a planner. Take stock of your commitments and assess what needs to be done. Examine your routine for any recurring flash-points (the school run and tea-time in my house...) then look for any ways to relieve the pressure.

Here's a personal example: Some days, the thought of an impending mealtime makes me want to lie down in a darkened room. However, if I'm honest, it's not the actual meal-assembly that's the hard work. More taxing is the wondering what on earth to make, or the wearying prospect of shopping for ingredients. But I've learned (the hard way) that a very small amount of forward-thinking makes a molehill out of this particular mountain.

As any Cub Scout will tell you, it pays to be prepared. Let's face it, you're going to have to do the work anyway - so which is better:

a disorganised frenzy of stress and panic, or a calm, preemptive strike? The ostrich approach or mañana attitude may be easier in the short-term, but at a price. You will pay later - in stress.

By reducing this and other energy-sapping episodes of rushing and stressing, you'll allow your natural vitality to emerge. So on that happy day, when your life is running like a well-oiled machine - you'll have bucket-loads of energy to enjoy it!

## Give yourself a break

When you're busy or overwhelmed, it's tempting to just keep working, even when your body is hinting that you should stop. However, foregoing rest periods, lunch breaks, even sleep, will not help you in the long term. Regular breaks are essential to keep you going, they recharge you, giving you renewed energy to see your jobs through. Not only that, taking a break will make you more efficient and productive. So, as contradictory as it sounds, by doing less you could achieve more.

You may have heard the phrase 'work smarter, not harder'. This philosophy works just as well within the home as it does in the workplace. So be smart! Take advantage of the well-documented benefits of regular breaks.

Taking a break suggests that you're in control, you're confident that there is enough time. This mindset alone contributes greatly to you actually *being* in control. But the real magic comes from you returning to your work refreshed and enthusiastic - you are then able to focus and prioritise. You will be more effective, so much so that you'll get the same amount of work done in less time - so your time out won't actually cost you at all.

Many successful people advocate power naps. They claim that these mini-sleeps have maximum benefits, ranging from more patience, less stress, better reaction time, increased learning, more efficiency and better health. Not bad for a quick snooze!

Even the Bible supports the idea. After a busy week assembling *a universe*, the Almighty scheduled in a day of rest. If even the All-Seeing, All-Knowing Creator needs regular break periods, what chance us mere mortals?

Besides, if you don't take voluntary rests, you may find that your body will make them compulsory. (Collapsing from exhaustion will cost you far more down-time than a managed breaks schedule.) When fatigue gets a hold, lack of energy can escalate to irritability, loss of concentration, a sense of helplessness, even pain - effects that take their toll even after you finish the work. And being exhausted not only makes small tasks seem more arduous, add to that the fact that you are far less productive. The result? You have to work harder for the same results, which makes you even more exhausted!

*The time to relax is when you don't have time for it.*

*Jim Goodwin*

So nip this downward spiral in the bud. Be sensible about what you can realistically manage, acknowledge what breaks you'll need to function well - then make sure you take them. You will be rewarded with increased energy, health, confidence and productivity.

So if you really want to get more done - take a break.

# Get sensual

You may have heard the phrase, 'You only get out what you put in.' Well, this applies to our bodies. If you want to get more from your body, it can reap dividends to pay attention to what you 'put in'. Although diet is one major aspect of this (more on that coming up), it's not the only way we can treat (or mistreat) our physical form.

Here are a few ideas of how to improve your flagging energy levels through less obvious routes - via your senses.

## Skin therapy

Did you know that skin is your body's biggest organ? Did you also know that what you put on or next to your skin can have powerful effects on your overall health, well-being and energy? So clearly, it pays to avoid unnecessary toxins or harsh chemicals in your personal products and, if possible, your surroundings. But as well as being defensive, what about being pro-active - is there anything we can do to give ourselves a boost, via our skin?

What if I told you there was something you could apply to your skin which would improve your circulation, increase your vitality, detoxify, strengthen your immune system and give you a healthy, youthful glow that will last all day? You'd probably expect such a treatment to come with a hefty price tag. But there's something that offers all these benefits and more - and it's free! Better yet, you most likely have unlimited access to it in your home, right now! So, what is this wonder skin treatment?

The humble cold shower.

Cold-water therapy is an age-old idea. The Spartans of ancient Greece would immerse themselves in cold rivers in order to keep fit. The ancient Samurai warriors believed that standing under ice cold waterfalls (or buckets of water) was a cleansing ritual that purified the soul.

On a purely physical level, a warm shower followed by a cold (or cool) blast improves the blood flow to your vital organs, with significant health benefits. It is also a tried and tested bonus to your beauty regime. The cold rinse is renowned for making hair stronger and shinier and giving your skin a younger, healthful glow.

And in terms of boosting your energy, cold showers can bring dramatic results. A brief cold-water blast at the end of your usual (warm) shower will leave you refreshed, invigorated and motivated to face the day. Not only that, these additional health and beauty benefits will boost your sense of well-being and encourage your natural vitality to shine through.

So how does it work? Well, the sudden change between the warm and cold improves the circulation to both your skin and your organs, including the brain. This can aid your mental health, concentration and even your mood. Although a warm bath or shower can be a useful remedy for low spirits or lethargy (water, in general, has a positive effect on your energy and mood) the revitalising boost of a quick cold blast serves to lift your spirits and invigorate your entire being.

Admittedly, a cold shower does not appeal to everyone. And the idea might struggle to tempt you out from a warm bed. But if you lack energy, it can be a powerful technique. Though it can be a shock, at first, it is undeniably invigorating, and that wonderful tingling-skin feeling is strangely addictive. But the idea is not to torture yourself. How cold you have your shower and for how long depends on what you're used to or can reasonably tolerate.

So if you'd like a free and easy way to look younger, feel better and increase your energy levels - brrrrave the cold. It may make you scream a little, but it should also make you smile a lot.

As a supplementary practice to the cold shower, dry-body brushing also has tremendous benefits - boosting your energy, circulation, health, beauty and vitality. The most commonly recommended technique to benefit from both of these easy methods is as follows:

★ Brush dry skin with a loofah/bristle-brush, before your shower

★ Apply almond oil to your body (for baby-soft skin!)

★ Shower as normal

★ Turn the temperature down (not too much at first...)

★ Wet feet first, then hands, then face

★ Gradually increase exposure and duration

★ When finished, wrap yourself in warm towels

★ Vigorously dry yourself

★ Rest for a short while, if possible

N.B. There are some occasions when cold water therapy may not be suitable, for example if you suffer from hypersensitivity to cold. If you have any health concerns or are in any doubt, always consult your doctor first. Also, cold showers are best avoided during menstruation. The effects are too harsh for the reproductive system at that stage in your cycle.

## Music therapy

Runners use it for rhythm. Spas use it for calm. Lovers use it for seduction.

Music is a powerful device. It can be used very effectively to alter our moods and our energy. You probably know this already, at least in theory. But often it can seem easier to just get on with the work (however miserably), without making the small effort to make it more enjoyable, i.e., putting on some great tunes.

Perhaps it's because music is so simple and easily available that its effect is overlooked or under-rated. But housework is a unique challenge - *anything* that can make it more bearable ought to be an integral part of the routine. So the next time you really cannot find the energy to tackle your domestic stuff - girl, put your records on!

If you can get into the habit of making music an essential part of the process - like putting on your rubber gloves - you will feel more motivated and have a much more pleasant experience. Many people find that housework is far less of a chore when accompanied by their favourite tunes. Not only that, when you add a fun or upbeat element to your essential chores, you tend to dread them less. This alone will free up all that energy that would have been lost bemoaning the inevitable.

Music washes away from the soul the dust of everyday life.

Berthold Auerbach

So why not make a compilation of your most-loved tunes to see you through your most-loathed tasks. Have a playlist specifically for cleaning which contains songs that make you feel energetic or that take your mind off the task in hand. Make sure you select songs that uplift you, though - if you are feeling down about the state of your house, you might want to steer clear of the lovelorn ballads!

★

Music is not the only aural solution to domestic tedium. Books-on-tape can make great companions to your domestic routine. Although they may do less to bump up your energy levels, if they help you approach housework more positively, they're a worthwhile addition. Personally, I've found audiobooks to be powerful motivators to do something mindless and repetitive. I've even been known to be so gripped by an audiobook that I seek out chores just so I can keep listening! (You can find my favourites in the Suggested Reading section at the end of this book or visit my blog at: www.makepeacewithhousework.com).

Audiobooks are also an ideal opportunity for some multi-tasking. For example, if you know you'll never get time to read that new novel, why not download the audio version and listen to a chapter a day as you go about your chores? (I once used several hours of *Pride and Prejudice* on CD to see me through a mammoth decorating session.) Or you could use your cleaning time as a chance to improve your mind or learn a new language.

I find audible.com to be the best resource for audiobooks. They have a membership scheme where you can get a vast range of titles at greatly reduced prices. They also offer a free trial, so you can try out the service at no cost. Alternatively you can usually get audiobooks from your library, for a minimal fee.

So why not make use of these audio tools, to boost your energy and motivation or to lift flagging spirits. They can be fun and effective motivators. And as your mind is exported to far-off lands, you will begrudge your housework less. Since you'll have something else to concentrate on, you'll experience less of that internal chatter about how boring and monotonous the work is. The result will be more enjoyment and less complaining - all via your ears!

Then, when your work is done, you can switch the playlist to 'easy listening' and enjoy a well-earned chill-out.

## Aromatherapy

Did you know that women tend to have a stronger sense of smell than men? This might explain why our menfolk are often oblivious to odours that we notice as 'unpleasant'. But if you do have a keen sense of smell, there are advantages and ways to turn smelly situations to your benefit. In the case of depleted energy supplies, the solution could be right under your nose...

Smells have power. They can stimulate our mood, provoke our memories and helpfully here, increase our energy. It may seem far-fetched that just sniffing something will restore our get-up-and-go, but our sense of smell is a fast-track to our nervous system. Our nasal receptors are in such close proximity to the brain (the olfactory nerve is the shortest of the cranial nerves), that smells have a rapid and acute effect on our mental state. The slightest whiff can provoke extreme psychological reactions, which can then affect us physically or emotionally. Ask anyone with a fear of hospitals how they feel about the smell of disinfectant. Or think of when you last smelled something that instantly brought back a long-forgotten memory. For me the smell of a brand new book will always take me back to childhood Christmases. (Thanks, Mum!)

> Nothing is more memorable than a smell.
>
> *Diane Ackerman*

Smells may be commonplace but their effects can be intense. Knowing which smells will make you feel revitalised, and then using them within the home, is a simple way to beat the energy blues.

The use of smells as remedies (aromatherapy) is not a new concept. The ancient Greeks and Egyptians used plant oils and spices to treat many of life's ailments. This practice is still popular in Eastern cultures today. In fact, some modern Japanese companies use the effects of smell to boost the efficiency of their work force, by diffusing the air in the workplace with aromas relevant to the time of day, (e.g., lemon in the morning to awaken).

Over the ages, our Western culture had lost sight of this powerful and accessible technique. However, aromatherapy is now enjoying something of a renaissance. Although yet to be endorsed by conventional medicine, it is regaining popularity with the general public - so much so that it's now relatively easy to get hold of good essential oils and aromatherapy products. That's good news if you're looking to reduce fatigue, because aromatherapy, for all its gentle and natural approach, can have powerful results.

Each of the many and varied essential oils used in aromatherapy have different characteristics and effects. Some oils are best for relaxation whilst others are renowned for their invigorating effects. Knowing which oil to use for which situation is part of the skill of trained aromatherapists. But to begin with, just knowing the most powerful effects of a few common oils will be a sufficient for home use.

As an energy-boosting starter-pack, any of the following have stimulating, reviving or invigorating properties (and many have the added bonus of reducing irritability and preventing headaches). If you have these already at home, just sniff out your favourites! Alternatively, a reputable store will often have samples for you to try. Regardless of the helpful effects of essential oils, you will gain optimum results if you actually *like* the smell. So to determine which will be the best for you - just follow your nose.

| | |
|---|---|
| Basil | Black pepper |
| Cardamom | Cypress |
| Eucalyptus | Grapefruit |
| Lemon | Lemon grass |
| Lime | Neroli |
| Peppermint | Pine |
| Rosemary | |

The properties of the above essential oils have many more uses than reviving flagging spirits. Most of the oils have a vast range of applications, ranging from medicinal to cosmetic. If you experiment in blending different oils together, you can create your own uniquely-perfumed natural remedies - so you don't have to be a celebrity to have your own signature scent!

On a less glamourous note, many oils can be used very effectively in home-made, eco-friendly cleaning aids. (For more details, see the Resources section at www.houseworkblues.com.)

Once you've chosen your oils, there are a number of ways of using them. Aromatherapy oils have traditionally been either massaged into the skin or inhaled. So unless you can find a willing masseur, here are some practical ways to introduce the aromas to your home environment (some of which are conveniently compatible with the domestic routine).

**As a room spray.** You can freshen the air in your home with natural, refreshing and deodorising scents. Adding a few drops of your chosen oil to water in a spray bottle makes a cheap and easy air freshener. By selecting energising oils, your rooms will not only smell pleasant but the scented air will quietly work its magic, helping you feel vibrant and revived. (Ensure your spray bottles are non-plastic, as essential oils can dissolve plastic which will then contaminate the oils.)

**As a drawer scent.** Add a couple of drops of oil to a cotton wool ball and place in a drawer/cupboard/wardrobe for pleasant and restorative whiffs as you put away the laundry. (Note: the clothes within will also absorb these scents, so if you intend to fragrance your family's cupboards - make sure it's an aroma they like!)

**In the vac.** For a zestful fragrance during the obligatory vacuuming, try this tip. Drop a little of your favourite energising oil onto a corner of newspaper, then vac it up! Then, whenever you vacuum, the air will be diffused with the refreshing and invigorating aroma.

**In the shower.** Add a couple of drops of oil to your bath or shower products, shake well, then use as normal. This is a quick and easy way to ensure you start the day feeling awake and invigorated.

Carefully selecting your essential oils and introducing them to your routine will do wonders for your energy levels. But aromatherapy is a holistic approach - it works to improve your overall health and well-being. So the benefit of this positive, healthy and natural therapy will go beyond increased energy. Used regularly as a refresher or general tonic, these powerful aromas can promote emotional balance, relieve stress and have therapeutic effects on both your mind and body.

Note: Essential oils can be very potent, and they have health and storage limitations. For example, some are unsuitable during pregnancy, some cannot be applied neat to the skin, and all are toxic if taken internally. If you'd like to explore aromatherapy further, there is a wealth of information freely available on the internet (www. quinessence.com is a great resource for information and products). Alternatively, many good reference books are available, including *Essential Oils* from the wonderful Neal's Yard Remedies (who also supply quality, reputable grade essential oils and products).

Armed with a little basic knowledge, aromatherapy can be a useful weapon in your domestic battle. So the next time you need a quick pick-me-up, forget the ill-fated caffeine fix and instead reach for nature's homegrown remedies. They will help to boost your energy, heal your ills and promote harmony between mind and body.

Oh, and they smell nice, too.

# Get out more

They say a change is a good as a rest.

So, one solution to poor energy levels is not to do less but to do *something different*. If you look around your home and all those chores just make you want to go to sleep (and I know that feeling), one of the most helpful things you can do is...go out.

You needn't go far. You needn't go for long. But even a brief respite can be a powerful energiser. Being surrounded by your chores can feel utterly draining. Escaping them will bring relief, so when you return, you'll feel more positive and capable.

For proof of this, cast your mind back to the last time you went on holiday - how did it feel good to come home? Did it look different? When you take a break from seeing the same things day in, day out, you come back with a new attitude. A new energy.

For many people, to forget the cares of work, they simply go home. But when your work is your home, and vice versa - it can feel as though there's no escape. This is particularly acute in those who stay at home, but for whoever does the lion's share of the housework, simply leaving the premises can bring some much needed perspective.

So the next time the state of your house is getting you down, go out! Even if it's only as far as your garden. In fact, weather permitting, the Great Outdoors is possibly the most powerful refuge. Reconnecting with nature, feeling close to the earth is good for your soul. It can recharge your life-force.

> Forget not
> that the earth delights
> to feel your bare feet
> and the winds long
> to play with your hair.
>
> *Kahlil Gibran*

Plus, you never know - when you get back, somebody else might have tackled the housework while you were out. (Miracles do happen...)

# Get happy!

Humans are natural pleasure seekers and there are few states more pleasurable than being utterly happy. So happiness is worth pursuing simply for its own sake. But there's another reason we should seek to bring more happiness into our lives - being happy is good for you!

Science is increasingly proving that happiness has physical benefits. When we're happy, we feel alive, joyous and optimistic. Aside from being enjoyable and an emotional boost, these feelings actually affect us on a cellular level. They actively contribute to our overall health and well-being, including our energy levels.

The health benefits are obvious when we recognise happiness as an antidote to that destructive modern phenomenon, stress. Chronic and prolonged stress is so detrimental to our health that experts believe it will soon be the Number 1 killer in the Western world. Since it's impossible to be happy and stressed at the same time, time spent in a happy state naturally excludes stress. But these 'happy times' have an after-effect, leaving you more resilient when stressful situations do occur.

Reducing stress unleashes more of your natural vitality - reason enough to pursue happiness. And according to Maxwell Maltz in his classic book, *Psycho-Cybernetics*, happiness can do even more. In a chapter devoted to the benefits of happiness, Maltz cites Russian psychologist K. Kekcheyev, whose scientific tests show that when humans are happy, we perform better. He even claims that when thinking pleasant thoughts, we see, taste, smell and hear better and detect finer differences in touch.

Psychosomatic medicine is even more proof of how a positive attitude affects our health. If you've managed to 'attract' Rhonda Byrne's *The Secret*, you will be familiar with the story of Norman Cousins. In *Anatomy of an Illness*, Cousins relates his recovery from a terminal condition - using *laughter* as medicine. He says, 'I made the joyous discovery that ten minutes of genuine belly laughter had an anesthetic effect and would give me at least two hours of pain-free sleep. When the pain-killing effect of the laughter wore off, we would switch on the motion picture projector again and not infrequently, it would lead to another pain-free interval.'

Cousins is not the first to suggest that positive emotions can cure our ills. In many Eastern cultures, poor health is treated holistically, rather than just medicating symptoms. Disease is viewed as a malfunction, a deviation from our natural state of wellness. The idea is that restoring our natural equilibrium, including emotional balance, will restore health. Ease is the treatment for dis-ease (disease).

The pursuit of happiness, then, is undoubtedly an investment in our health, well-being and, subsequently, our vitality. But it's not only a boost to the quality of our lives right now, it also improves our chances of longevity - meaning we'll have more years to be happy in! So as a tool to increase energy levels, happiness is useful, but as an approach to a long and enjoyable life - it's essential. (This is even without noting other 'happy' side effects such as increased wealth and productivity...)

*N.B.* Although happiness can improve your health and your sleep, it can be hard to 'get happy' if either your sleep or health are lacking.

> Nobody really cares if you're miserable, so you might as well be happy.
>
> Cynthia Nelms

It's a chicken and egg situation - but if you can crack it (pardon the pun) your efforts will be rewarded. If you can get into a cycle of good sleep/good health/good spirits, your energy levels will skyrocket. And your life will be a lot of fun, too!

## So, how do we get happy?

You may now be thinking, *This is all very well in theory, but finding happiness is easier said than done.* You may even be thinking that you'd love to be happy, but can't until the necessary circumstances arise, e.g., you come into money, find your life partner, have perfect health or your dream career, etc.

In answer to this I would suggest there are two routes to happiness. Route A is the hold-out-for-the-perfect-life scenario. You postpone happiness until everything that you believe will make you happy arrives. The downsides of this method are: a) those circumstances may never arrive; b) by the time they do arrive, you may have changed your mind; c) the longing and pining of the wait is not much fun; and d) you miss out on all the joy along the way.

Route B, however, has a bit more going for it. Route B is the DIY route to happiness. The instructions for this are coming up, but first, the benefits: a) *you* are in control, b) you get to experience happiness *right now!* c) the 'work' involved is absolute bliss!

So, what exactly is the DIY route to happiness? Well, it's actually a very simple 3-step process.

## Step 1: Discover your power

When we realise exactly what happiness is, we also find out who controls it. So, time to ask - what is happiness?

Happiness is an *internal response*. Though it may often be influenced or provoked by external effects, it's *our interpretation* that gives rise to happiness. This explains why two people can see the same person/object/view, and one can be indifferent, yet the other is enraptured.

So it's not outside circumstances that dictate whether or not you will be happy. A good example of this is money. Many people believe money will bring them happiness, yet some rich people are miserable, whilst some with little money live very happily. Similarly, housework is neither good nor evil (stay with me...) - some hate it but believe it or not, some love it! The emotion comes from inside, from our reaction, not from the work itself.

Reacting happily (or unhappily) is often an unconscious response based on what we believe about ourselves and our happiness. But our internal reactions can be guided or controlled. With practice, you can direct your internal thoughts and responses. You can literally train yourself to be happy! Which means *you* are in charge of your own happiness. It's not necessary to wait for your circumstances to change. Happiness is not something that happens *to* you. You control it.

So, how do we begin this process? How do we reclaim command over our own happiness? It starts, very simply, with the intention to do so. Instead of waiting for *other things* to make you happy, or letting *other things* stop you from being happy - you can choose to be happy, regardless. It's possible to make a conscious choice to be happy, whatever the circumstances.

It sounds far too easy to be true - but just try it! It really works. Should you intend it, you can choose to be happy despite what's going on around you. In this way you can make happiness a habit, rather than an occasional treat. Of course, like any new habit, it may require considerable effort at first. And there may be times when you simply can't manage it. But don't give up. It will gradually get easier and in time will be your natural response. And it's a habit that will change your life.

(Just as a personal tip: I find it helpful, on days when I'm struggling to stay upbeat, to believe in The Grand Plan. I take much comfort in the idea of a benevolent force that has our ultimate good at heart and has got it all in hand. So even on the 'bad days', I can relax, knowing that all is as it should be. Even if you're not wholly convinced by this theory, as a consideration, it can reduce the angst and disappointment which can be a feature of everyday life.)

So it's your attitude, your response or happiness-habit and not circumstances that make you happy. For further evidence of this, have you ever come across someone who you considered unfortunate or poorly done to, yet they appeared remarkably happy? I once went into a particularly dark and dingy public toilet (I was desperate!) where I encountered the cleaner. I don't think there can be many people who would have envied her job, yet she was one of the happiest souls I've ever seen. I was amazed that she could be happy at all in such a place, let alone, whistling and smiling. This lady had cracked the skill of being happy, regardless. Her happiness came from within and it was powerful enough to overcome her external circumstances.

*The habit of being happy enables one to be largely freed from the domination of outward conditions.*

*Robert Louis Stevenson*

Whilst it's true that some people are blessed with a naturally sunny disposition, for those of us who aren't, there's still hope. Every one of us has the potential within to live happily - some may just have to work at it a bit harder. For many happy people, their happiness comes from a conscious intention combined with regular practice.

Now you may protest, *How can I possibly choose to be happy with my circumstances? How can I ever find happiness until so-and-so does x, y or z?* But these are self-imposed limitations. Whilst it's true that we can't force other people to meet our criteria - we can choose to change our criteria!

Here's a personal example. I used to believe (given my feelings about domestic work) that I could never be happy unless I had a cleaner. I was wrong. I've since experienced unhappy times whilst having a cleaner, and happier times when I didn't. My criteria were wrong - I discovered I could actually be happy without my self-imposed limitations.

Just as it's possible to be unhappy even in pleasant circumstances (think of miserable rock stars, for example), it's also possible to be happy in unpleasant conditions. However, if your situation is particularly dire and you are certain you cannot be happy, what about just being *happier*?

The pursuit of happiness is not about being ecstatic every minute of the day. Dr John A Schindler defines happiness as 'A state of mind in which our thinking is pleasant a good share of the time.' This is realistic, and a reasonable goal. Besides, without the contrast of occasional unhappy times, we wouldn't appreciate the pleasant times as much. The lows make the highs more valuable. This is not to say you don't try to improve an unhappy situation. But equally, don't pin all your happiness on those future improvements.

> Most people are about as happy as they make up their minds to be.
>
> *Abraham Lincoln*

Be realistic; accept that everyday life has its challenges. But to make your experience of life a happier one, remember that you control your happiness. You may not be able to change your circumstances, but you can decide how you will react to them. Happiness can be a choice. And the choice is yours.

## Step 2: Know where it exists

It's impossible to experience anything in the future. We can't feel happiness, or any other emotion, in any time other than the present. Yet many of us tend to postpone our happiness until some future date, when everything will be 'just right'. But how likely is it that such a day will ever arrive?

It's true that there is much pleasure to be found in dreaming and planning and setting goals. In fact, it is only natural. Humans are goal-striving beings, at our happiest when pursuing a goal. However, the pleasure comes from the thinking/dreaming/planning that *occurs in the present moment*. Though you may, in the future, improve your life, it's not necessary to wait until then to enjoy it! Your life doesn't have to fit a certain criteria for you to be happy - unless you decide that.

So why wait? If you take the time to stop and look around, right now, you may find you can enjoy the journey as much as the destination. Perhaps more! Besides, when you get whatever you're waiting for -

then what? Will you be completely satisfied? More likely, there will be something else you want but don't have. Look at those people who literally do have everything - are they satisfied? Some of the most successful people in the world are also the most driven - constantly chasing the next idea or goal. This is the nature of life - a constant forward motion. But if you wait for the finish line before you enjoy it, it will be too late!

If you ask yourself *Where is my life right now?* the answer will probably be: *I'm doing quite well in this department but there is work to do here.* This will always be the case! There will always be some aspect which is good and there will always be something that could make you happier - but why not take comfort in this? The acceptance that you will never be completely satisfied, never 'finished', can be an enormous relief. It highlights the futility of delaying your pleasure and joy. It means you might as well relax and enjoy life now.

All you need to do to be happy now, is: a) be aware of your present circumstances and b) focus on the best bits. Practice recognising more of your existing happiness. Again, this is a habit which can be easily formed with intention and repeated effort. Soon it will be a natural reaction - and with powerful results. When you spend more time focussing on your present joys, not only do you become more positive, generous and *happy*, but according to the laws of physics (what you focus on expands) you will be increasing the things that make you happy - in the present and the future!

For every person, without exception, there will be something good in their present moment. Perhaps it's just the roof over your head, or that your children are safe and well, or even the mere fact of being alive. The key is to slooooow down and notice.

> Happiness is a mental habit... and if it is not learned and practiced in the present moment it is never experienced.
>
> Dr Maxwell Maltz

For example, we often race through a delicious meal, barely tasting our food. Or we might hurry past a beautiful landscape or sunset, focussed on future worries and missing the awe-inspiring spectacle around us. Nature has an enormous capacity to stimulate joy and happiness which is freely available to everyone - all we have to do is remember to look.

Learning to recognise and appreciate the positives in your life, *this very moment*, is a surefire route to happiness. Give it a go! In fact, why not try it now? Look around you and notice where you are, how you feel. Keep looking until you see, hear or feel something that makes you smile. And there you have it - happiness now. It was there all along.

So, by all means have an optimistic eye to the future. Keep dreaming, planning and imagining a better life, as that is a joy in itself. But remember to enjoy the thrill of the chase and find the fun in where you are. Decide to find your happiness *right now* and you always will.

## Step 3: Be proactive

Though you can develop the habit of being content with any circumstances and finding joy around you, there are times when you won't need to try at all. Welcome to your bliss! Your own personal bliss is whatever causes you to smile, or sigh with happiness or jump for joy. Your bliss occurs naturally, without effort or conscious intent.

When we regularly make room for these occasions of happiness, the result is a healthier, calmer, more energetic and agreeable version of ourselves. Your bliss is good for you! With the busyness of modern life, these pleasures often get squeezed out of the schedule for 'more important' things. Yet this is short-sighted. It serves us to value whatever brings us joy - and do more of it!

> Sometimes your joy is the source of your smile, but sometimes your smile can be the source of your joy.
>
> *Thich Nhat Hanh*

If the results of our happiness are so hugely beneficial, clearly we should be actively pursuing what makes us happy. The first step in doing this is to recognise your own personal source of bliss. Discover what floats your particular boat. Just considering this will raise your awareness. When you discover what makes you happy or what you believe will make you happy, make room for it in your life. Upgrade its importance. Do more of whatever brings you joy. *Follow your bliss.*

Start small if necessary. For example, if you feel utterly at peace with the world during a massage - book one! Schedule them on a regular basis. Women often dismiss their pleasures as 'optional'. But now that you realise the importance of following your bliss, what are you waiting for? Maybe shopping is your personal pleasure. If you have the means, don't wait for permission from anyone else. Certainly don't feel guilty. Your sheer enjoyment is justification enough.

Once you're on good strong terms with your bliss, there's more you can do to promote you happiness even further, through a process called 'amplification'. All this requires you to do is really enjoy your happiness! Revel in it. When you find the things that bring you joy, however small, amplify your good feelings. The effects of being conscious of your happiness are a powerful double-whammy. Firstly, you increase the physically boosting effects that happiness brings. The happier you are, the better for your overall health, energy and well-being. Secondly, science dictates that what you focus on, particularly with strong positive emotions, will grow. Which means more occasions for you to feel this happiness!

But is it selfish to so eagerly pursue our own happiness? No! You are, indirectly, doing the world a favour. To totally neglect your own needs is a recipe for misery - and a miserable you is not great for those around you. Plus, a compelling feature of happiness is the wish to share it. Think back to the last time you were in a great mood. You probably wanted to share your joy with others. You smiled more at strangers. You were more willing to help or to give. In short, you had a natural urge to spread the happiness. Being happy makes us naturally selfless. Compare this spirit of generosity with those who sacrifice their own joy.

Whilst it is true that there is much happiness to be found in the service of others, this needn't exclude your own needs. Begrudgingly offering your services has little value, whereas serving others joyfully in addition to following your own joy is a win-win scenario. So don't be afraid to indulge in whatever makes you smile. Regularly.

## And finally...

So, there you have it! The 3-step route to happiness. You now know the reasons to choose happiness, and how to do it. In theory, this knowledge should be enough to ensure a blissful life experience. In reality, though, however reasonably the head's argument, sometimes the heart will call the shots. Some days, for no particular reason, you're just in a slump. You're human. It happens. So, for these occasions, you'll need to bypass logic and go straight to emotions.

Cue my Top Ten Emergency Uppers...

**1. Look for the silver lining**. However bad things are, there's always something positive you can focus on. If it's any consolation, there will always be someone worse off than you.

**2. Find clues in your blues**. If things are getting you down, that's a clue to what would bring you up - so focus on that. Collect images of how you would like things to be. Select pictures or photos of your ideal situation. If the state of the house is depressing you, look at pictures of beautiful interiors. If your children are driving you mad, look at a photo of them being angelic and adorable.

**3. Know your rescue remedies**. Make a list of all the things that always make you smile, no matter how low you go. It could be books, places, people. Look for the sparks, those little gems of life that always bring a smile to your face. Only you know what they are.

**4. Treat yourself.** *Make* the time.

**5. Call the Blues Police**. Be alert for bad moods and notice when you are getting grumpy or moody. It's much easier to snap out of the blues before they get a hold. Try to spot any patterns of bad moods. For example, if you get tetchy on certain days of your cycle, you can take vitamins or make changes to your diet. Or if the morning rush puts you in a foul temper for the day, search for ways to help life run more smoothly.

**6. Play that tune**. Music is a powerful mood booster. It's hard to feel gloomy with your favourite song in your ears. Even better, sing along - loudly! It will raise your spirits and your energy levels, and it's fun!

**7. Eat, drink and be merry**. There are certain foods that stimulate happy chemicals within our bodies. Chocolate is the obvious one. Weigh up your nutrition/weight goals with the effect of unhappiness. What you gain in calories, you may burn off with increased vitality and joy. However, there are less calorific options. Did you know that brown rice has antidepressant qualities?

Drink, used sparingly and responsibly, can also be helpful in offsetting a downward spiral. We all need a little something to take the edge off a bad day. However, practice caution - a glass of wine may soothe your worries, but a bottle may increase them!

**8. Go naturale**. Getting out in nature gives us perspective. Our misery somehow pales in significance when we consider our place in the grand scheme of things. Mother Nature has the capacity to heal our hearts and soothe our souls. Naturally.

**9. Breathe**. Getting more oxygen into our lungs calms us both physically and emotionally. So, get a good lungful of air, the fresher the better. Breathe deep. And be happy that you can.

**10. Keep a good sense of humour**. Often the things that really get to us would actually be quite funny - if they were happening to someone else! The ability to laugh, despite everything, is a powerful skill. It's a fast-acting Blues-Blaster but it will also keep you healthy and youthful. And smiling.

# Let's get physical

Housework is physical work. Although this book is mostly focused on the psychological aspects of your domestic schedule, all of that's irrelevant if you're not physically fit and able. Keeping a home can be an endlessly demanding task. You are going to need stamina. So, if your goal is to conquer the domestic realm, it pays to keep yourself in good shape.

## Fitness first

Regular physical activity will improve your fitness, which will naturally increase your energy levels. Of course, with our busy modern lives, that can be easier said than done. As self-defeating as it can be, our health and fitness plans often have to take a back seat to our many other commitments. Women, selfless creatures that we are, tend to put the demands of work/home/family before our exercise regimes. (I know I am guilty of this - my beloved yoga sessions regularly get postponed or cancelled as something 'more important' crops up.)

But neglecting our fitness is short-sighted. Lacking the energy to competently meet our commitments is not in the best interests of our loved ones - or ourselves. So, the answer is to re-prioritise. Choose your favourite form of physical exercise, whether it's swimming, pilates, or tree-walking, even just a daily stroll. Then assert its place in your routine. Make it non-negotiable.

You are not neglecting your family in doing this. On the contrary -

*The first wealth is health.*

*Ralph Waldo Emerson*

you're ensuring their upkeep by maintaining the workforce (i.e., you). And as any manager will tell you, when the workforce is operating below par, it is inefficient (not to mention miserable). So, any steps that you take to boost your physical energy will benefit your home and family. Being physically fit will ensure you have the energy to cope with their demands.

## Many Birds, One Stone

Ensuring a place for exercise in your schedule will work wonders for your energy levels. But this exercise time needn't always be at the expense of something else. When faced with a multitude of people and tasks clamouring for your attention, a little multi-tasking may be in order. For these occasions, there's a way you can squeeze in your exercise time whilst *simultaneously* meeting your commitments...

Instead of viewing housework as part of the problem (too much to do, not enough energy, no time to exercise...), if we're clever, we can use it as the solution. Allow me to introduce the multi-faceted benefits of...The Housework-out! Housework as exercise. It's the perfect multi-tasking occupation. You get your chores done whilst improving your physical fitness.

And housework is a totally legitimate form of exercise. Walking up and down stairs is a great aerobic workout. Chores such as vacuuming, dusting and mopping burn almost as many calories as walking at a moderate pace. More intense tasks such as spring cleaning, gardening and chopping wood are even better for physical fitness.

Viewing your chores as 'potential work-out aids' is a far more positive approach than begrudging and/or avoiding them. The active nature of most housework will automatically increase your energy levels and help keep you in shape. Polishing, dusting, mopping and sweeping are a good upper-body work-out, firming those upper arms. And all that bending, twisting, reaching and stretching is great for toning thighs and waists. Plus, building up muscle can really help with weight issues, since muscle burns more calories than fat - even when resting! So turning your chores into your work-out will not only get you feeling more naturally vibrant, it'll keep you looking in good shape, too!

But can the simple domestic schedule really do all this? Like all forms of exercise, the more effort, movement and energy you put into your work, the more health benefits you will reap. (Aim for 20+ minutes of a raised heart-rate for aerobic benefits.) Plus, the little and often nature is perfectly in line with current medical advice regarding exercise. And since housework is less intense that some sport or gym workouts, you are less likely to injure yourself. Not only that, one major side-effect is that you regain control over your domestic workload and have a clean and comfortable home for you and your family to enjoy. And it's free!

All this makes The Housework-out a multi-result activity. In addition to the benefits to your home and physique, housework has also been proven to be beneficial to your mental health and emotional balance. So you will also reduce those energy-sapping episodes of stress or depression. Any form of exercise encourages the release of endorphins into your body. These happy chemicals improve your mood and provide an emotional boost. This experience is pleasant, enjoyable and, believe it or not, can become addictive - you may have heard of people becoming addicted to the gym. Although I don't advocate you become addicted to housework, knowing that it's good for your physical, mental and emotional health, your home-life and life in general, may just help to motivate you mop-wards!

## Break the cycle

At this point you may be thinking, *That's all fine in theory, but doesn't help if I can't find the energy to get started!* Admittedly, breaking the cycle of lethargy and inertia is tricky. This is because you're caught in a nasty catch-22 situation: the idea of the work is depressing which depletes your energy even further, giving you less energy to tackle it. (Not to mention any negative feng shui chi lurking in the 'neglected' areas...)

But it's well worth making the initially tough effort of breaking this cycle because it would spark an upward spiral towards better health, increased energy and a home that feels more like a sanctuary than a sweat-shop. So if this is enough motivation, the best way to tackle it is to start small.

Chances are, the work surrounding you didn't occur instantly. It built up over time. And so it can be reduced the same way. Taking small, gradual steps is probably the best tactic if you're really struggling to get started. Knowing that vacuuming the entire house will make you feel energetic may not be enough of a motivation for you to even get the vac out. So just plan to vacuum one room. Or maybe just tidy up so that you can vacuum tomorrow.

I appreciate that, at first, it can be really hard to get the momentum going, so as an extra motivation, be aware that any small energy-boosting step you take will be *triply effective*, if you use that energy to tackle a little housework. For example, if you decide to go for walk to pep up your energy, this small, simple exercise will make you naturally more energetic. If you then use this energy to do a little light vacuuming - you'll stir up some new fresh energy within your home. The positive effects of this will increase your energy levels even further. You will also reduce the angst of worrying about the vacuuming. Not only that, the physical exertion involved in vacuuming will increase your energy levels even more! It's a triple whammy - you reduce your stress, boost your health and improve the positive energy in your environment.

Hopefully, the promise of these gradual results will help to motivate you to get started (take heart that it will only get easier). Once you've begun, however, another useful idea to keep in mind is this: *just keep going*. There will be days when you feel you just don't have the energy - but don't give into that idea! If it occurs to you, you can choose to disagree. In the words of that great World War II poster, 'Keep Calm & Carry On'. Expect occasional lapses, accept them as *temporary* blips. But don't allow them to make you give up, because any momentum you've gained will be lost. Then you'll have to start from scratch again, which is even harder. Be encouraged that as your energy levels increase, these lapses will be fewer and farther between.

> Movement is a medicine for creating change in a person's physical, emotional, and mental states.
>
> *Carol Welch*

In case you still need convincing of the merits of The Houseworkout, here's a summary of the many, many advantages and benefits *to you*.

★ Nobody is likely to complain that you are selfishly taking 'me-time'

★ Your new-found energy makes the workload easier

★ The positive effect of getting the work done is a psychological boost

★ It's cheaper than a gym membership

★ You don't need to travel

★ Your home will become a nicer place to be

★ You will feel less/stressed/depressed/overwhelmed by your domestic workload

★ A clean and tidy home has a positive effect on your natural vitality

★ Your family will think you are a domestic goddess and worship you accordingly

Choosing housework as your regular exercise will undoubtedly improve your energy levels. You'll be fitter and more able to manage both the physical and mental demands of maintaining a home. And the more you do it - the better you'll manage.

But the real magic is that by the time you've worked up some energy, your chores will already be done! So you can use all your extra energy to go out and enjoy life. You'll have both the time and energy to pursue the life you want - beyond housework. Plus, when you get home, your house will be spotless.

Now that's a bonus you don't get from the gym.

# Quality Essentials

Breathing, eating, drinking and sleeping are the four essentials of life. These are the invisible foundations on which our lives are built. When our foundations are strong, we cope better with whatever the world throws at us. When any of these essentials are lacking, life can be unnecessarily tough.

We can control the quality and quantity of these four elements. Yet, because they are commonplace, even unconscious, their power and potential often get overlooked. But with a little knowledge, attention and intention, we can ensure our core infrastructure is sound and supportive. The result will be naturally high energy levels alongside a more productive, successful, enjoyable life.

Time to get back to basics.

## Breathing

Breath gives us life, we all know this. Beyond this fact, though, we often don't give breathing much thought. Our subconscious mind very helpfully takes care of the details, which is fortunate - can you imagine if we had to plan every breath! Yet what we breathe, and how we breathe, can have an enormous impact on both our physical and mental health, and our energy levels. So it may help to give this simple act a bit of conscious consideration.

### Deep breathing

Take a deep breath. In.....and out. Easy, isn't it? Yet it's one of the fastest and most effective tricks for boosting energy. Plus you can do it anywhere, anytime - and it's free!

When you breathe deeply, into your stomach rather than just your chest, you absorb more oxygen. This is a rapid energiser, but you will also benefit from increased focus, concentration and circulation, lower blood pressure and reduced stress. All from just a tweak in your breathing technique.

Your breath is a powerful tool. It is literally your life force. Taking the time, just occasionally throughout your day, to focus on your breathing can really help to restore your vitality. And it's a great device for emotional balance, too. (Just try it the next time you feel beaten by the Housework Blues...)

Though there are many intricate and complex techniques to using breath as a tool for health (explore yoga for more on this), you can still enjoy enormous benefits by keeping it simple. And what could be simpler than breathing? So, go on - do it again. Inhale. Exhale. Ahhhh.

**Good air**

The quality of the air you breathe affects the quality of your life. Anyone who suffers with airborne allergens will appreciate the effects of what we inhale. It has both the potential to harm (think fumes, pollution, toxins) or to heal (think of the old cure of 'taking the sea air'). Ensuring we get regular doses of good-quality air will benefit our energy levels, our overall health and even our mood.

It pays then to consider the atmosphere, wherever you spend most of your time. If you can, takes steps to make the air as healthful as possible. For example, our modern centrally-heated, double-glazed homes may be warm - but how fresh is the air? Just opening a window can usher in a life-enhancing dose of fresh air that can really make a difference to your personal energy and the energy in the home.

Also, if you have electrical equipment in your environment, these can drastically reduce air quality. As we have increasing numbers of electronic devices in our homes and our lives, the damaging effects of electromagnetic frequencies (EMF) are becoming a major concern.

Luckily, Mother Nature offers a quick and easy remedy to offset some of this, in the form of the humble houseplant. Peace lilies are particularly effective at neutralising the negative emissions of computers and TVs, etc. Even if you are hopeless with plants (like me), they are still a worthwhile investment in your health. View them as a fleeting pleasure, like fresh flowers. Even if they last only slightly longer than fresh flowers, in their brief life they will happily replenish the air in your home and the quality of your energy. Plants are great for mopping-up undesirable ingredients in the surrounding air. So, even for the really hopeless plant-carer, it's better to have limited success with houseplants than no houseplants at all.

Beyond the air in your home, though, nothing beats going to a place of naturally good, clean, invigorating air - in a forest, beside the sea,

> For breath is life,
> and if you breathe
> well you will live
> long on earth.
>
> *Sanskrit Proverb*

on a mountain top. Anywhere the air is naturally pure has revitalising properties. So for a great health, energy and well-being boost, take a fresh-air pilgrimage whenever you can. Seek out quality air and breathe in the benefits. Both body and soul will thank you for it.

## Eating

If you had to be a meal - which one would you prefer to be: A lovingly-prepared bounty of fresh, chemical-free produce? Or a ready meal?

Given the choice, few would opt for the latter. But the truth is - you are a meal! In fact, you are every meal you've ever eaten, at least in part. It's a cliché that 'we are what we eat', but it is fundamentally true. Our bodies convert whatever passes our lips into the very stuff we're made of. As a result, every aspect of your physical self may be influenced by the food you eat.

*Tell me what you eat, I'll tell you who you are.*

*Anthelme Brillat-Savarin*

Food is energy. So, if your energy levels are lacking, food can provide the remedy...or be the culprit. Your body can only convert what you give it. The quality of what you put in will affect what your body gives you back. Any body will struggle to manufacture vital exuberance if it is only ever fed life-less, nutrient-less junk.

Without a doubt, your energy levels affect your ability to maintain your living space. An exhausted person will tolerate much more mess and chaos than an energetic one. (I can vouch for that...) So, although you may not often state: *I can't cope with housework because I eat the wrong foods*, there could well be a connection between your diet and the state of your home. Your food - your fuel - affects your energy which affects your home, and consequently your life.

This is ironic, since the state of your house can often be a catalyst for a spot of comfort eating! It's the old catch-22 situation. But recognising the link is an effective step in the right direction. Knowing that what you eat will have repercussions can guide you towards a more supportive diet.

For example, if you suffer from fatigue, it helps to know that refined sugar is not your friend. I speak from experience. I once went to see a diet specialist who, naturally, quizzed me about my food choices. She casually declared that I had a 'sugar habit'. 'What!' I protested. The odd biscuit? (or cake... or chocolate...etc.) I wasn't addicted!

I could stop at anytime... She was right, though. Over the following days I monitored my reaction to sugar and realised that at a certain time *every day,* I literally craved it. I couldn't think of anything else. If I was out, all could think of was getting home to my tea and cake. It was my refuge from life. Some turn to alcohol or work or drugs. My crutch was a big bag of flapjacks.

However, I also noticed that after my 'fix' of the 'white poison', the only thing I then wanted, quite desperately, was to lie down and sleep. I believe that's called 'crashing'. I decided that this was no way for a healthy adult to function. My food choices were literally sapping my life away.

I share my woeful tale, but not as an indictment of all sweet goods. (I believe the world would be a miserable place without our chosen treats and indulgences.) My point is that being aware of the effects of what you eat is empowering. You can make diet decisions based on understanding. You can change *when* you eat certain foods to cushion the side effects. You can control how you will feel, or at least explain it (or, in the case of children and ketchup – you can be prepared for when the sugar kicks in!). Instead of wondering why you have no energy, you can find clues by monitoring your diet. This may or may not motivate you to make changes in what you eat, but at least it will be an informed decision.

> To eat is a necessity,
> to eat intelligently
> is an art.
>
> Francois de La
> Rochefoucauld

The role that food plays in our lives is often underestimated. I believe we can help ourselves (and our children) to a better life by exploring it. There are many great books and resources about eating your way to health, vitality, even youth! (My current favourites are: *Yummy!*, *Body Foods for Life*, and *You Are What You Eat.*) Arming yourself with this knowledge is a powerful step towards your goal of vibrant energy levels.

A healthy, informed relationship with food does not mean denying yourself the enjoyment of food. In fact, it's likely that the opposite may occur. By being more aware of the quality of what you eat, and focussing on when and how you eat, you'll probably find that you actually enjoy food more! So be smart, be informed, take control. Eating well is a recipe for living well.

Bon appetit!

## Drinking

Sometimes an energy slump is not a result of underlying health or lifestyle problems. It may just be down to what we've done on that particular day. Or in the case of drinking enough water, what we *haven't* done.

We all know the drill - drink at least eight glasses of water a day. Yet it can be tricky to enforce this, if you're not in the habit. The solution? To get into the habit! Managing to get enough water into your daily routine is one of the best things you can do for your health, well-being and vitality. It can even give you a beauty boost!

Our bodies are approximately two-thirds water. We need to replenish our daily supplies to ensure our bodies function properly. If we fall short, even only slightly, our body reacts with emergency measures, which range in severity from mildly unpleasant to very serious, even fatal.

Symptoms of mild dehydration include

- Lethargy
- Irritability
- Depression
- Poor concentration
- Headaches, migraine
- Impaired sleep
- Dry skin
- Joint problems, arthritis
- Sore eyes
- Digestive problems, constipation, heartburn

Of course, some of the above may be symptomatic of other health issues, so an easy way to see if you're dehydrated is to have a wee check in the loo. Literally. If your urine colour is any darker than very pale yellow - get yourself a drink!

Recognising the importance of water for quality of life is a good motivator to ensuring you drink enough. But to make it easier, try to adopt one or two of the following habits. Then, when they become second nature, try a couple more.

★ In social settings, alternate alcoholic drinks with mineral water. You'll barely notice at the time but you'll be very thankful the morning after! (Also helps with weight loss.)

★ Keep a bottle of water and a glass on your desk and by your bed. You're more likely to drink it if it's within easy reach. Plus it's a visual reminder. Note: Beware of keeping drinking water in plastic bottles in the car or in the sun - the heat destabilises the plastic and can make the water toxic.

★ Alternate herbal tea with your daily cuppa. There are some great herbal teas widely available. These not only provide you with more water but have health-giving properties themselves. (I love Dr Stuart's and Pukka's delicious, nourishing teas - not least due to their cool packaging!)

★ Instead of reaching straight for the painkillers when you get a headache, try a glass of water first. It could just be your body trying to tell you that you're dehydrated.

★ If you get bored of water on its own - mix it up! Combine a good quality fruit juice half-and-half with sparkling mineral water for a refreshing long drink (helps towards your fruit portion too!)

*Our bodies are molded rivers.*

*Novalis*

The current guideline for quantity is two litres throughout the day (avoid drinking large volumes all at once). It's important to increase your intake in hot weather, if you are exercising, or if you feel lethargic. The above tips can help you meet your body's needs with very little effort. In fact, you may only notice the difference when you get through the afternoon without yawning - or when somebody compliments your glowing complexion!

Ridding your life of those niggling minor ailments and unleashing a new vitality with glowing natural beauty to boot - all from the humble H2O? Let's drink to that!

## Sleeping

Sleep is essential for life. So much so, that sleep deprivation can be fatal. Although most of us will manage to get enough sleep to live, do we get enough to live *well?*

Increasingly in our hectic society, sufficient sleep is viewed as optional. When life gets busy, sleep is often the first thing to be sacrificed. But this is a short-sighted solution. A more beneficial response would be to prioritise sleep *more*. By making adequate sleep non-negotiable, you will be healthier, have more energy, be more efficient, more capable and less stressed.

By recognising how vital sleep is for our health, and how it impacts the quality of our waking hours (poor energy is a common indicator of inadequate sleep), we will be more likely to give it the priority it deserves. So it pays to be aware of the restorative powers of sleep. For all its appearance as a passive, inactive state, there is much essential maintenance work going on under the surface...

The beginning of health is sleep.

*Proverb*

During this rejuvenating down-time, our bodies recuperate and our minds sort through the barrage of thoughts from the day, attempting to make sense of them all. We need this regeneration work to function optimally. Without it, our health, emotions and mental abilities begin to deteriorate. We literally malfunction. Some common effects of sleep deprivation are fatigue, daytime drowsiness, weight gain, premature aging, irritability, and slower mental reactions.

It's clear, then, that getting enough sleep is important. But how much is enough? This is tricky - even the experts can't agree. Though the general consensus is that a healthy adult needs 7/8 hours a day, that is only the average. Your own personal needs will be affected by factors such as age, weight, diet, habit, genes, gender, lifestyle, etc. If you are unwell, you may need to sleep more than normal. (There is much truth in the old idea that sleep is a great healer.) If you've accumulated a sleep debt, you may also need more hours than usual.

However, contrary to popular belief (and logic), weariness isn't always due to a lack of sleep - it can actually be the result of sleeping *too much*. Many people claim to feel lethargic and slow after their weekend lie-in. If you feel sluggish and apathetic, yet you regularly get more than 8 hours a night, try 7. It sounds perverse but try it for a week or so and see how you feel. The added bonus of this is an extra waking hour in your day! (Whether you inform your family you have more free time available is up to you...)

Probably the best way to find your own optimum requirements is to monitor your sleep patterns and how they make you feel. Professor Jim Horne, Director of Loughborough University's Sleep Research Centre says, 'The test of insufficient sleep is whether you are sleepy in the day or if you remain alert through most of the day.'

However, it's not just the quantity of sleep that affects our energy levels, health and faculties. The type of sleep we get is important too. It's a case of quality, not just quantity. Lack of *sound sleep* can decrease your quality of life and accelerate the aging process. Fatigue and daytime drowsiness can be a result of too little of the restorative deeper phases of sleep. It is during these phases, when our brains produce delta waves, that our bodies replenish and heal. Melatonin is released, along with other hormones that repair and regenerate tissues, build bone and muscle, strengthen the immune system, and reduce aging.

Whether you need to get more sleep or just better quality sleep, there are many tricks you can use to help improve your slumber. For example, an obvious tip, if you drink a lot of alcohol or caffeine, is to try cutting back, especially close to bedtime. Also, regular exercise has always been a great, chemical-free remedy for inducing sound sleep. Fresh air, particularly sea air, has a gently sedative effect (and also anti-depressant qualities!). And a good quality bed and bedding are an investment which will reap dividends in the quality of your sleep.

A good laugh and a long sleep are the best cures in the doctor's book.

*Irish Proverb*

Also, don't forget that the winding-down time which is such a vital part of an infant's routine, is equally relevant to adults. The combination of regular bedtime, subdued lighting and relaxing, non-stimulating activities such as reading, taking a bath, perhaps adding a little lavender oil to your pillow, all act as powerful signals to the body that it is time to sleep. It's also widely regarded that a lack of electronic items in the bedroom is more conducive to better sleep.

Arming yourself with this sleep info may give you a big advantage in your battle against fatigue. Obviously, if you have a sleep disorder, these simple techniques may be inadequate (although they may help a little) and fatigue may be a symptom of something other than lack of adequate sleep. But for the average weary person, prioritising sleep and ensuring the quality of your down-time will do wonders, not only for your energy levels, but also for your health, mental abilities and general well-being.

Note: For anyone needing to recharge but unable to ensure more or better sleep (insomniacs, parents of young children, shift-workers etc), there is another option. Although sleep undoubtedly provides the most comprehensive overhaul, good old-fashioned R&R comes a close second. Some organs and muscles can be regenerate in a relaxed, restful state, even if you're not asleep. So, if you really can't sleep, don't fret too much (this may actually be more harmful than the lack of sleep). Take heart that by simply resting, your body will still gain restorative benefits from a relaxing time-out.

Alternatively, consider the Power Nap. Sleep expert Professor Jim Horne suggests that most people would get more out of a 15-minute afternoon nap than an extra hour of sleep at night!

So listen to your body and respect what it needs. And if it's telling you to have a quick snooze, it just may know what's it's talking about.

# Go with the ebb and flow

The human body is a robust and resilient thing. It's able to survive unimaginable trauma. It has an immense capacity to heal itself, even from supposedly life-threatening conditions. But it is not a machine. As a natural, organic entity, it is subject to the laws of nature. It is prone to the way of the universe: ebb and flow.

Everything in existence moves in cycles or waves, from the planetary orbits of the solar system to sub-microscopic particles. Our bodies are no different. For example, we are all subject to the cycle of birth-life-death. And on a day-to-day level, we've evolved to follow the cyclical calendars with their patterns of days, weeks and years.

Whether we like it or not, these cycles affect us. Admittedly some people feel it more than others, but we're all subject to the cycle of the seasons and our 24-hour day. And though we all have a natural reserve of vitality, these too are subject to cycles. There may be times when flagging energy is the result of nothing more than a natural dip.

Some cultures work with these natural energy peaks and troughs. The afternoon siesta is typical of hotter climates - yet it would suit many of us, regardless of the weather. But even if the society in which we live is not a perfect match, there's still much we can do on a personal level, once we begin to recognize our own cycles and patterns.

## SAD but true

A recent medical phenomenon is that of Seasonal Affective Disorder (SAD). It's now widely recognised that some people are *biologically affected* by the onset of winter. Symptoms include mood changes, lethargy, food cravings, even depression. Some patients are even prescribed medication. Increasingly, though, light therapy is an effective and popular solution. But perhaps the most helpful step is in recognising that you are affected. Then you can try to adjust your life to your natural flows.

On a personal note, I believe I've been affected by SAD. I once spent an utterly miserable winter, beset with chest infection after chest infection. I felt like the most unhealthy being on the planet, a condition made even more painful by my goal of being fit and healthy. Many visits to doctors revealed nothing helpful. I hated all the medication

I was prescribed, which prompted an all-time low of sobbing and wailing, 'I just want to be well!' I was just about at the point of despair, when spring arrived. My symptoms magically began to disappear.

As I learnt more about the healing power of sunlight, I regained full health. Since then I have survived a number of winters with my health intact. Armed with my new awareness, I take steps to ensure I have the strength to deal with the darker months. Health has become my priority and I actively aim to boost my immune system and general health. And at the first ray of winter sun, I will be outside, basking in it - despite the temperature!

Some people are so severely affected by SAD that they migrate to sunnier places during the winter months. Others adjust their work schedule, or at least the type of work they accommodate during their 'low season'. Though not everyone has such control over their home or workload, even small changes to your personal life can relieve the struggle. For example, if you are naturally inclined to hibernate in winter - ease up on the social calendar. Or if you feel the loss of regular sunlight, plan your beach holiday to break up the duller months.

> Every mile
> is two
> in winter.
>
> *George Herbert*

By becoming aware of how you're affected by the natural seasons, you can accommodate your body's needs. This will help you stay in harmony with your natural tendencies rather than forcing yourself into an unnatural pattern. And by eliminating any unnecessary struggle, you will cope better with natural energy dips.

## Larks and owls

Similarly to our seasonal rhythms, we all have our own internal clock which controls our energy throughout the day and night.

We're all familiar with the circadian cycle of 24 hours a day and in our Western culture, the typical working day is from 9am to 5pm (ish). But not everyone naturally suits that cycle. Some people are night owls, at their best in the evening. Then, there's their polar opposite - morning people, who like to be up early and do half a day's work before the rest of us are out of bed.

Neither of these types is necessarily better, as such. Since we are all different, what suits one may be disastrous for another. But what the larks and the owls have got right is their awareness of their own rhythms. If you are struggling with a lack of energy, it may be useful for you to try and discover your own rhythms.

This awareness can be very helpful if you then seek to manage your life with it in mind. When you work with, rather than against, your natural rhythms, you'll find success and achievement more effortlessly. So, not only will you be in harmony with your energy cycles (thus more energetic), life will naturally be less of a struggle.

For example, if you are at your most effective in the early morning, yet have a lifestyle where you stay up late (and hence rise late), you'll be less effective later in the day. If you miss your lively, productive mornings, you may be falling short of your potential. Yet this does not mean you're an ineffective person. It just means your life is operating out of sync with your natural energy peaks and troughs.

As much as you can control your activities, you'll be doing yourself a huge favour by, firstly, monitoring your natural patterns, and secondly, adjusting your life accordingly. For example, I have a friend who claims she does her best work in the hours when her family are asleep. This means she needs an afternoon nap but since that fits into her day, it's not a problem. Working in harmony with her rhythms, she produces work she is proud of whilst managing her family commitments.

So if you want to unleash more of your natural energy resources - know your patterns! Monitor when you feel naturally energetic, when you are alert and able to focus. This way you can plan the relevant activities for that time of the day (or night).

Admittedly, we are limited in how much we can control our timetable. As members of society, we do have to fall in with certain social schedules. (Although supermarkets may now be open at 3am, the dentist almost certainly won't be!) Yet the changes that are within your power, even though they may be small at first, are a step in the right direction. And discovering and honouring your body clock will effortlessly release more of your innate vitality.

## 28 Days

As well as the human sequences of days and years, there's another biological cycle which is uniquely female. The monthly one.

In our modern culture, there are no allowances made for women during menstruation. We're expected to carry on as normal. It has even become politically incorrect to acknowledge differences in female physiology. Yet, women's bodies do undergo significant biological changes during the menstrual cycle.

You may wonder how a book by a self-proclaimed feminist could concede such a thing. But I don't believe that being equal is the same as being identical. Whilst I would argue for gender equality, I would stop short of insisting that men and women are the same. Physically at least, we are subject to a whole different system of hormones and their subsequent effects. To be discreet about this may be more socially acceptable, but it helps no one if we deny it to ourselves.

So what are these 'differences' that we are sweeping under the carpet? Well, some *normal* symptoms of menstruation are: pain, cramps, headaches, bloating, diarrhea, fatigue, PMT and anaemia. Although severity varies between females, even the more minor effects can have a significant impact on our ability to function normally. And some women suffer from severe symptoms for a whole week, every month. That's nearly a quarter of their child-bearing years! Quite a considerable length of time to be operating below par. So the least we can do is acknowledge these regular changes within our own bodies.

I recently came across the idea that women ought to rest during the first couple of days of their menstrual cycle. This had never occurred to me before. The reasoning was that the significant loss of blood and vital nutrients that women experience on a monthly basis required (and justified) a spell of R&R. Although this is not the generally accepted view, it actually makes good sense. If a person lost the same amount of blood under less regular circumstances, e.g., accident or illness, they would be prescribed immediate bed rest! Yet because the menstrual cycle is a predictable and commonplace feature, we're expected to pretend that it has no effect on our bodies.

> Feed a cold.
> Starve a fever.
> Give PMS
> anything
> it wants.
>
> *Unknown*

And the loss of blood is not the only significant effect. The fluctuation in our hormones can powerfully influence how we deal with life. Though, again, women are affected to varying degrees, none of us are immune to hormonal changes. After all, if these hormones had no effect, why would the body produce them? Yet we often dismiss these imbalances, as if to admit to them would somehow be a weakness. Many women who believe in equality may balk at expecting special 'women-only' treatment. But surely to deny our unique biology is a bigger disservice to our sex.

Perhaps many women feel they wouldn't be taken seriously if they asked for 'lighter duties' during their time of the month. The sad truth is that they would probably be right. Studies suggest that women are viewed less positively, even as less capable, during their period. This is a far cry from the ancient view that women were miraculous creatures who can produce life from their loins and bleed without dying! In modern times, the 'time of the month' is a little more taboo. Even though this function is natural to the female body, it's often labeled as a curse and treated as an affliction.

The unspoken solution to this modern lack of empathy is simply to keep it to yourself. However we can, and I believe should, make our own quiet and private acknowledgement that we need a temporary phase of rest, gentleness and taking care of ourselves. So, if your schedule is within your control, ease up on the workload. You needn't inform anyone of the reasons why. (Women can be shrewd and wily creatures, able to stealthily advance our own ends - why not make use of that skill?)

> Women complain about PMS, but I think of it as the only time of the month when I can be myself.
>
> *Roseanne Barr*

After all, a time of restfulness is our instinctive response, developed over millennia of physical evolution. Modern timetables may make it inconvenient or social politics may deem it inappropriate, but our bodies don't know all that.

This is a special period (pardon the pun). You owe it to yourself to at least recognise that you're undergoing physical, psychological and emotional changes. Your body needs to adjust and for this it needs you to just lay off a bit. Instead of trying to struggle through or medicate the symptoms, why not embrace your femininity and give yourself a break?

Even if your workload is beyond your control, your leisure time is under your jurisdiction. Use it to accommodate your body's need for rest. If you neglect your me-time for the rest of the month, make sure you at least indulge yourself a little for these few days.

## Know thyself

To reclaim your innate vitality and enjoy improved well-being, get on friendly terms with your natural cycles. Discover your own rhythms and tendencies, your personal peaks and troughs. Then you can make decisions based on that knowledge. When you know how *you* work, when you can anticipate your highs and lows, you can plan accordingly. If you're expecting a lull, you can go easy on yourself, knowing it's only a natural blip. Or if there are times when you have to battle through a low-energy time, at least you'll know to implement your emergency energy boosters - before the lethargy gets a hold.

Working against your natural rhythms makes life unnecessarily difficult. So it pays to become aware of your own unique patterns. Instead of battling through demanding tasks when you are in a cyclical downturn (e.g., PMT), you can aim to structure your life to go with these flows, instead of using all your energy to fight them.

This is the easier option - yet it's also the most productive. For example, if you force yourself to work through a time when you're physically exhausted - how effective will you be? If possible, why not wait until you're full of beans and can whizz through the same task with a fraction of the effort. This will save you time, energy and stress. Dr Deepak Chopra calls this 'The Universal Law of Least Effort'. He says, 'It's based on the fact that nature's intelligence functions with effortless ease and abandoned carefreeness. The principle of least action, of no resistance.'

So ease up on the struggle where you can. Find your flow, then go with it.

# Toxic home

Although your home may be the victim of your lack of energy - could it also be the culprit?

According to the World Health Organisation, 'sick building syndrome' can occur in the home and has a disruptive effect on performance, relationships and productivity. Lethargy and tiredness are recognised symptoms.

Sick building syndrome is essentially any negative health effects that arise from being in a particular building. It's mostly associated with buildings that were constructed using harmful products or those with serious damp problems. However, the combination of double glazing, central heating and inadequate ventilation make for poor air quality in many modern houses, which can greatly impact the health and vitality of the inhabitants.

A potentially greater concern, though, is the emission of toxins or the out-gassing of chemical-laden products that we bring into our homes. So even if a house itself is not harmful, the contents may be.

Whilst this information may be alarming, there's no need to panic - most people can cope with a degree of toxins in the home. We humans are generally quite robust. However, if you suffer from inexplicable lethargy in your home, it may be worth considering the healthful/harmful aspects of the building you live in. And regardless of your current health, it's also worth learning about the potentially harmful aspects of some everyday products.

Knowledge is power.

*Frances Bacon*

One of the best things you can do initially is insure adequate ventilation. Beyond that, arming yourself with knowledge will enable you to make informed choices about what you allow into your home.

To start you off, here's a brief list of 'areas of concern':

★ Pressed wood (MDF, particle board, etc). This is glued together with formaldehyde and can continue to emit these fumes in the home, though the fumes are sealed by painting. It is commonly used in ironing boards and furniture.

★ Paint fumes. When you decorate, you can usually smell the paint fumes. They may even give you a headache. This is because the fumes contain potentially hazardous substances. They can affect the air even when the paint has dried. Luckily, less harmful paints are becoming popular and easily available.

★ Air fresheners. These may mask odours (or coat your nasal passages so you can't smell them) but the chemicals contained in some leave the air anything but fresh. Many contain known toxins, including potential carcinogens. (Home-made air-fresheners are a relatively easy to make and cost-effective alternative - plus you can be sure what's in them.)

★ Carpets. These often contain glue which can emit air pollutants called 'volatile organic compounds' (VOCs). Although this off-gassing diminishes after a few months, it can continue for years.

★ Fly spray. Insecticides contain poison - that's how they work. There have been concerns, however, that the chemicals don't just harm the insects but could be carcinogenic when inhaled by humans.

★ Electrical items. Electromagnetic frequencies (EMF) are emitted by electrical appliances and power lines. Electromagnetic radiation (EMR) is emitted by most wireless devices and microwaves. Although the jury is still out on the potential harm from these frequencies, there is definitely cause for concern, or at least caution and awareness. Suspected symptoms are: the disruption of natural energy levels, an increase of the stress response, and a higher incidence of certain diseases.

★ Cleaning products. This is possibly the worst offender when it comes to toxins in your home. Although it would be ironic if your cleaning products are making you too lethargic to clean your house, it could actually be the case. Many commercial cleaning products contain harmful chemicals. Some ingredients are so strong that inadvertently mixing them could prove fatal.

Please note, the above list is intended to highlight products with *potentially* harmful ingredients. Increasingly, there are paints, air fresheners, cleaning products, etc that don't contain harmful substances and it is certainly worth doing a little homework to seek these out.

It's also true that not all pollutants in the home are man-made. Some biological pollutants (i.e., from living organisms) can also be harmful to your health. Again, another symptom of this kind of pollution is fatigue. If you're particularly sensitive or allergy-prone, it may be that dust or mould spores are affecting your health. (This is another instance of catch-22: not cleaning robs you of the energy you need to clean. But don't despair! Instead, spin this fact around and use it to motivate you - keeping your home spotless will result in more energy, enabling you to effortlessly keep your home spotless!)

Regardless of the source of any pollution in your home, there are some simple steps you can take to tackle it. Although there are many good books dedicated solely to this topic (see Resources at www.houseworkblues.com for more details), here are a few quick examples of what you can easily do to improve matters:

★ Ensure good ventilation. Open windows regularly to aerate your rooms.

★ Introduce an air purifier, either electronic or natural (e.g., Himalayan salt lamps).

★ Make use of the natural air-cleansing properties of houseplants.

★ Use a vacuum with a HEPA filter and vac regularly (sorry!).

★ Get a large doormat and/or operate a 'no shoes' policy.

★ Swap synthetic cleaning products for more natural alternatives, e.g., lemon, vinegar, baking soda, salt, etc. (*The Humble Art of Zen-Cleansing* is a great little guide to using these.)

If you think you may be under attack from the hazardous effects of modern living, be aware that air is not the only way toxins get into our bodies. For example, our skin is the largest of the body's organs, and anything applied to it can make its way into our system.

This is of particular concern to women because of some of the ingredients in beauty products. It is also relevant to parents who apply products to their children's skin. (I was shocked to discover that some baby oils are petroleum by-products.) Again, the shift towards natural baby and beauty products is encouraging. These are increasingly available and reasonably priced. (Although even if there is still a premium for these products, weigh up these extra pennies against the cost and misery of ill-health.) A favourite resource of mine is the wonderful LoveLula. This online store sources products that are ethical, natural, organic, eco-friendly and of course, utterly gorgeous.

(They also send free samples!)

Another invisible way we accumulate toxins is in our diet. People are increasingly opting for organic or home-grown produce - and with good reason. Developments in mass-producing our food may have progressed at the expense of our long-term health. We're increasingly learning of the detrimental side-effects of modern food production and there may still be effects of chemical or artificial treatments that we're yet to discover. The only way you can be sure of the provenance of your food is by buying direct from reputable suppliers, buying organic or growing your own. Admittedly these options sometimes have a time or financial cost but at least you know you won't be paying with your health. (Plus the pleasure to be had from home-grown fruit and veg is not to be underestimated!)

Some of this information may be shocking and perhaps a little frightening. But I share it not to induce panic, rather to highlight potential hazards that may be sapping your energy or health. It's impossible to live in the modern world and remain unaffected by its dangers, but forewarned is fore-armed. Awareness and education are your strongest allies. Once you know the dangers, you can take steps to reduce them or seek out more healthful alternatives.

> Forewarned, fore-armed.
>
> *French proverb*

Doing a little research can also unearth more reassuring information. For example, if the contents of your house are quite old, they have probably stopped emitting gases and fumes. Also, very recent items are likely to be much less harmful than those from earlier years.

Fortunately, we're experiencing a social shift towards more natural, environment- and human-friendly products and processes. Consumers are wising up and rightly wanting to protect themselves, their families, their homes and the planet. As a result, eco-credentials have become an effective marketing device. Green is fashionable and what people want, businesses will provide. There's a definite trend towards more holistic and wholesome products and processes. It would be nice to think that these companies' decisions to opt for less harmful routes is ethics-based and not solely profit-driven, but ultimately what matters is that we now have a choice. It may currently be a more expensive one (though the gap is shrinking), but it's a step in the right direction for all of us.

Whilst it's encouraging that the reckless degradation of both our personal and global natural resources is (slowly) abating, there's still a long way to go. Our supermarket shelves are still packed with products that contain a frightening list of dubious ingredients. So while you are waiting for the world to catch up, take your health and vitality into your own hands. Be aware of what you allow into your home and your body. Empower yourself with knowledge. And if any of these ideas strike a chord with you - investigate them further. It could be that your famous feminine intuition is trying to tell you something...

# Clutter-bust

Do you have clutter? You're in good company, if you do. It's a common modern problem. More and more of us are becoming inundated and overwhelmed with 'things', drowning in our own possessions. But the normality of this clutter habit belies its insidious and damaging nature. Clutter is more than unsightly pockets of stuff that need sorting out. It's an energy-drainer. Clutter can drag you down, both mentally and physically. Declaring war on your clutter will reap innumerable benefits, not least of which will be a boost to your energy.

Clear and uncluttered spaces are restful to the mind. In contrast, having too much stuff is mentally unsettling. Your mind constantly scans and evaluates every item, reminding you what needs to be done with it. Your home is meant to be a refuge from the world, a place of calm where you can retreat from the bombardment of 'stuff'. But when your home is also packed full of 'stuff', your mind gets no respite, no chance to recharge. Facing this on a regular basis can be exhausting, leaving you poorly placed to face to world outside your door.

So, clutter costs you your mental energy, but that's not all. There are emotional and even physical effects. Aside from the depressing effect it has on your natural energy, clutter makes you irritable and stressed, which drags down your mood even further.

In feng shui terms, clutter is stagnant energy. According to this ancient wisdom, our homes have an energy of their own which naturally circulates and flows... until it hits a clutter pocket. Here it gets stuck, and just as water stagnates when it cannot flow, this energy (known as chi) becomes negative and oppressive. The effects of this range from fractious relationships to unnecessary struggle, even to poor health. Your clutter can literally make you ill.

However much faith you have in Eastern ideology, there are benefits to de-cluttering that can't fail to convince even the most cynical Western minds. For one thing, you'll spend less time searching for

> Clutter causes stress, and is one of the main barriers of productivity.
>
> *Charisse Ward*

things. In studies on clutter and untidiness, the time spent frantically tracking down misplaced items can amount to hours! That's far more time than it would have taken to tidy up in the first place. Secondly, when your home is tidy, you feel proud of it. This is a boost to your self-esteem (with all the ensuing benefits). Thirdly, in an ordered environment, there's less visual and mental distraction - you can think more clearly. And finally, you have somewhere you can relax, which is vital for good health and psychological well-being.

Also, according to finance expert Suze Orman, decluttering is a route to more financial success. In her best-selling book, *Women & Money*, Suze claims that one of the 8 qualities of a wealthy woman is cleanliness, or the need for order and organisation in your affairs. She even goes so far as to say 'when your car looks like a garbage can, when your closets are filled with junk and clutter, I'm sorry but you can't possibly be a wealthy woman.' According to Suze, if your affairs remain a mess, wealth will elude you. This may sound harsh, but then, do you know any millionaires with a clutter-problem?

A place for everything, everything in its place.

Benjamin Franklin

Perhaps the most compelling argument for de-cluttering, though, is that housework is difficult enough! Clutter makes keeping the place clean *much* more arduous. Not only does it take longer - when you're faced with a mess, you're usually less inclined to do it. And with flagging energy levels, you'll feel even less able to tackle it. For example, vacuuming is a great way to freshen up the stale energy in the room, but it will be less effective and more labour intensive in a room full of clutter. So, if for no other reason than to make housework easier, cut your clutter!

Keeping a clutter-free home is very simple. There are two basic rules: Have a Place for Everything and Put Things Away. However, simplicity does not equal ease and sticking to these rules can be tricky, especially when other people are involved. You'll have to come to terms with the idea of constant and never-ending effort. It's an ongoing battle. The only way you can win is with a ceaseless 'little and often' strategy. And it doesn't matter where you start, only that you do - and that you keep going! Whatever mountains you have to face, by constantly chip-chip-chipping away, you will eventually reclaim your home. And once you do, stay motivated by remembering that keeping on top of clutter is much easier than tackling it when it's got a hold.

This is another instance where forming a habit will help you immensely. By training yourself to *automatically* pick up things that are out of place and to get rid of unnecessary items, you'll be well-armed in the defence against clutter.

If you're truly determined to take control of your clutter, there are many books, websites, even TV shows that will help and inspire you. You can even hire professional declutterers. Many of these offer varying methods, so go for whichever appeals to you. Personally, I find little in common with naturally tidy people sharing their tips. I prefer the ex-clutterers who have converted.

> Out of clutter, find simplicity.
>
> *Albert Einstein*

The ones who dug themselves out of their clutter-nightmare - I can relate to them. One such author is Cynthia Townley Ewer and her book *Cut the Clutter* is an inspiring and entertaining read. And my current 'virtual clutter mentor' is Mimi Tanner, whose eBook and course *Declutter Fast* have proven very motivating. (She cites the comforting advice that 'Clutter is finite!')

So face up to your clutter. Take it on. You can win this war. It may not be a breeze and there may be days you want to give in, but if you persevere - the rewards are considerable. Plus the more you do it, the easier it gets.

Eliminating your clutter is a powerful step to making your home a more healthful, energising and supportive place to be. And I speak from experience - when I first clutter-busted a very chaotic dining room, I actually felt a noticeable shift in my energy. Even other people commented that the room 'felt different, roomier, *lighter*'. So, I can't stress strongly enough that being clutter-free is truly worth the effort. (Can you spot the convert?)

Keeping your home in order will leave you less stressed and more naturally vibrant, confident and in control. So form a healthy intolerance for any clutter invasions. Then, like the good healthy chi circulating happily round your home, your life will flow along more nicely, too.

Section 5:

# boredom

How could we possibly be bored within the home? There is so much to do!

Yet the term 'bored housewife' is prevalent for good reason. In the domestic realm, boredom arises not from a lack of things to do - there is usually a multitude of chores awaiting our attention. The trouble is finding something *we want to do*, something that excites or stimulates us. When it comes to housework, all too often the prospects are tedious or dull or uninspiring. Boring.

So far, so familiar. But there are actually a number of ways of dealing positively with boredom. For instance, it can be helpful to accept that a degree of boredom is inevitable. Similarly, learning to turn boring activities to your advantage can also be a useful trick. And since prevention is always preferable to cure, this section also includes ideas to nip feelings of boredom in the proverbial bud.

First, though, it may be useful to examine the nature and consequences of boredom, to find clues on how best to tackle it.

## The nature of boredom

Humans have a natural love of variety. So when boredom arises, from a lack of change or variation, we get twitchy, and seek out new, more stimulating options.

Unfortunately, housework, by its very nature, is a series of repeated actions - the same tasks done over and over. It's the same house, kitchen, clothes, etc that need cleaning repeatedly, endlessly. Our brains soon get used to these sights and actions, and we get bored.

So take comfort in the fact that, as an intelligent human being, you will be bored by mundane and repetitive tasks. Anyone with a modicum of intelligence would be crying out for a bit of variety. It is natural and understandable.

## Boredom - good or bad?

Housework is boring, no news there. What might be helpful to consider, though, is whether that is necessarily a bad thing? Some of the ideas that follow will show how mindless, repetitive activities can actually be beneficial to your physical health, psychological well-being, and even your creative success. Instead of fighting boredom, it's actually possible to exploit the mundanity of obligatory tasks to improve other aspects of your life.

A degree of boredom, then, is not only inevitable but potentially good for you. The key thing to note here though is 'a degree of boredom'. An *excess* of boredom is another matter. There are good reasons to reduce feelings of melancholic boredom - they are not only dispiriting, they can be hazardous to your mental health. Boredom can be dangerous. It can be the start of a downward spiral which progresses to existential anxiety (a sense of *What's the point...?*) and eventually, depression. When boredom turns from mild domestic tedium to a severe or debilitating apathy, it ought to be taken seriously. Extreme cases are unlikely to be caused by the dullness of daily maintenance and may be a symptom of something more serious. (At which point, professional or medical help may be required, and the sooner the better.)

> Boredom
> is rage
> spread thin.
>
> Paul Tillich

Happily, though, there are steps you can take within your home and domestic schedule to relieve everyday boredom and make sure more serious problems don't get a hold. If you are veering towards an overload of the monotonous and the mundane, it's possible to reduce feelings of ennui by simple tweaks of your attitude. Boredom is perception-based, i.e., all the angst is in your head, arising from your view of the problem. Considering a new less frustrating perspective can provide much relief.

There are also practical steps you can take to counteract thoughts that lead to boredom, little tricks to liven up the monotony. Although some tactics may require extra effort, in battling boredom, our priority isn't to avoid work, but to make it less psychologically frustrating. Taking extra steps purely to relieve boredom can be well worth the effort.

So given that boredom can be both good and bad - should we encourage it, tolerate it or avoid at all costs? I believe the ultimate solution to be a collaboration of all three approaches: accept a certain amount, reduce where possible, and make use of what's left.

And for the hows and whys to do just that? Read on...

# Now for the boring bit...

Between the ups and downs of life, there will be the boring bits.
(Hopefully you won't find this section to be one of them...)

OK, you're bored. What do you do? Resent it? Fight it? Avoid anything that bores you? Boredom is a void which we naturally try to fill or replace with something more inspiring. Some of the time, this is what's required - but there are occasions when it'll do you more good to just go with it.

Boring, mundane, uninspiring activities are an unavoidable part of life. Coming to terms with this idea will benefit you in two ways. Firstly, it will prevent you battling in vain against an inevitable truth. The universe is based on a system of ebb and flow, highs and lows, ins and outs, intense experiences followed by spells of down-time. So learning to accept some boredom as a naturally occurring part of life will bring you less angst and more serenity. Knowing it's only a temporary state can be something of a comfort, too.

Secondly, giving yourself permission to accept a little boredom takes the pressure off you to cram every second with stimulating activities. Everybody has some element of their life that they find boring or tedious - and this is a good thing! Can you imagine how exhausted you'd be if you were permanently challenged or excited? Life can be pretty hectic these days - boredom can be a welcome pause from stimulation overload.

So instead of instantly feeling resentment when you find yourself bored - allow a little. If you can meet boredom with a calm acknowledgment of 'yes, this is boring but that's fine, it's not forever - it's just an oasis of down-time in the busyness of life', you will be making great strides along the road to enlightenment, serenity and fewer frown lines.

# Worse things happen at sea...

...or, indeed, on land.

The next time you're wiping the table after what feels like the millionth feeding frenzy (or whichever chore is your personal boredom-bugbear) and you're struck by the utter boredom of the task, just hold that thought. Don't worry, I'm not going to try and convince you that there is joy or stimulation to be found (I'd struggle on that score). However, I am going to suggest that 'boring' is not the worst thing a job could be.

I doubt poultry processors, hospital clean-up crew, morticians, or terrorist negotiators would cite boredom as their main complaint - but would you want to swap roles with them? When I begin to contemplate the dreary, mundane nature of certain unavoidable tasks (pairing socks is another one, yawn....) I find it helpful to remind myself that at least I am warm and dry. I'm not battling traffic, dealing with a tyrannical boss, being abused by irate customers or facing extreme danger.

> Mayhem achieved, boredom relieved.
>
> *Bruce McCall*

To consider the plight of those with more unpleasant or treacherous jobs can be a useful tool in offsetting boredom. Yes, your task may be mind-numbing, but try to look on the bright side - at least, within the home, you are your own boss, the conditions aren't too unsavoury and the risks to life and limb are minimal.

## Diamonds in the dust-heap

Just as an aside, looking on the bright side is a powerful attitude shift which can benefit every aspect of your life. (Did you know, optimists tend to live longer?) Finding the positive is not always easy, but it does get easier with practice. So the next time you are faced with your most yawn-inducing task, use it as an opportunity to improve this vital life skill. Look for the diamond in that particular boring dust-heap (there's always something).

Once this technique becomes a habit, it will not only improve your sanity (and your home) but will also reap numerous benefits for your health, wealth and happiness, too!

# Get your kicks

Housework sometimes gets a raw deal. Is it possible that we blame housework for frustrations which actually stem from dissatisfaction in other areas of our life?

Admittedly, if things in general aren't going well, housework is more likely to get you down. But that doesn't necessarily make it the main culprit. In bemoaning the boredom of housework, you could be seeking excitement and stimulation in the wrong area of your life. Housework is maintenance. It has its benefits and can even be therapeutic, but its primary purpose is not to entertain and amuse you.

So if you regularly feel beset with utter boredom in your domestic chores, instead of trying to make mundane tasks more interesting, discover what does excite and stimulate you - then do more of that!

Live it up - beyond housework. Whether that means travel, hobbies, friends, career - you know what floats your particular boat. You'll then return to your jobs feeling more fulfilled and less resistant to any essential but boring work. (This tactic also reduces the crippling analysis of the worthiness of housework, which is a torment all of its own.)

If you are living a full, exciting and challenging life, then by the time you have to face those mind-numbing chores, you might be ready for some down-time. You may even welcome a stint of mindless unchallenging activity. However, if you come to realise that it's *your life* that's lacking in stimulation and excitement, at least you now know where the true problem lies - which is often the first step to solving it.

So you are hereby required to go out and enjoy yourself. In pursuing what makes you happy, you will naturally become less reluctant and thus more effective on the domestic front.

Life and housework in perfect harmony - who'd have thought it?

# An Attitude of Gratitude

Oprah is a fan. *The Secret* raves about it. It's featured in many self-help guides and success manuals, including centuries-old classics and the Bible. And if you take only one idea from this book, I hope that it's this one:

Gratitude.

It's a small, easy, commonplace sentiment, summed up in two little words: thank you. Yet it's a powerful tool which can transform your life. I believe that this concept, more than any other insight in this book, will not only improve your domestic situation but will affect your whole life. Quite a bold claim! But I am utterly convinced of the simple power of an attitude of gratitude.

Where does this power come from? What are the effects? And more importantly, how can we harness it to cope with the boredom of housework?

## The Power of Thank You

So how does it work? How can simply being grateful affect your life? There are a number of theories, some spiritual, some scientific, and there are many books dedicated solely to this topic. However, it's a simple principle, so a brief explanation is all you need to see how it can work for you. (Though if you feel drawn to gaining a deeper understanding, *The Secret* book/film or the *Wealth Beyond Reason* resource are great places to start.)

As diverse as the many explanations are, they all agree on one thing: An appreciation of what's good in your life will bring more good things to you.

Gratitude is a classic example of the idea that what you focus on, expands. Spending time, thought and energy on any aspects of good in your life is a powerful act of focus. This conscious appreciation shapes your perspective, you become more positive, more optimistic, helpful, and joyful. This new attitude affects your approach to life and subsequently, your results. It's an upward spiral that attracts more things into your life to be grateful for! Who wouldn't want that?

According to John Assaraf, author of the best-seller, *Having It All*, when we count three blessings a day, we get a measurable boost in happiness that uplifts and energizes us. And former US television anchor Deborah Norville focuses on the scientific evidence of the gratitude factor in her book, *Thank You Power*. Deborah claims that gratitude can make you healthier, happier, smarter, more resilient, and can even undo the negative effects of stress.

It makes psychological sense. When you consciously seek the silver lining, you're literally training your brain. Whatever you give thought to, your brain is programmed to notice more of the same - have you ever been considering buying a certain car and you strangely start noticing the same car all over the place? Well, when you consider what's wonderful in your life - you suddenly start to notice even more wonderful things. The Law of Attraction explains this phenomenon by suggesting that gratitude makes you magnetic to more of what you're focussing on - in this case, more good stuff!

When you are thankful, you're acknowledging your blessings and good fortune - even if only in small ways. This state of mind leads you to becoming more blessed and even luckier. Quite a result! And it all begins with a sense of appreciation.

## Gratitude versus Boredom

How does all this relate to being utterly bored with housework?

Allow me to use a personal example to show how gratitude can obliterate domestic boredom: I used to have a big problem with making beds. I found it futile, monotonous and utterly boring. Yet I love a nicely-made bed, so I'd grumble through the chore, every single day. Then one winter, I found myself on the cold streets of Edinburgh, with some people from a charity for the homeless. They were doing a publicity stunt, a Sleep-Out. On the streets.

I joined them for a while (though not all night) and it was a rude awakening to the harsh, freezing reality of homelessness.

Since that day, I use my bed-making as a reminder to be thankful that I have a warm, safe and dry place to sleep. When sparing a thought for others who may not be so lucky, it feels petty and spoilt to complain about a job that, although repetitive and unchallenging, takes only a few seconds of my day.

The following quote sums up beautifully how this gratitude attitude can offset the tedium of the domestic routine:

I am thankful for a lawn that needs mowing,
windows that need cleaning
and gutters that need fixing
because it means I have a home.
I am thankful for the piles of laundry and ironing
because it means my loved ones are nearby.

*Nancie J. Carmody*
*(in Family Circle magazine)*

It's also possible to harness the power of gratitude within the home as both prevention and cure of boredom. It's difficult to focus on two things at the same time, so if you concentrate on what's good in your life, that leaves less brain-space to think about any boring bits. Plus, if you are in a positive and thankful frame of mind, you'll be more accepting and less resentful of the obligatory mundane tasks. So the boring bits will bother you less.

Add to this the attraction factor (i.e., you get more of what you think about), you'll soon be attracting more stuff to be grateful for and less stuff that bores you. Beware of the downside of this theory, though. Ingratitude, or focusing on all that's wrong, e.g., boring, with your situation will, guess what...? Bring you more of the dross! Even more reason to switch your focus towards gratitude.

## Small domestic mercies

So if you'd like to give this quick, easy and powerful technique a try, here are some domestic applications to get you started. Try the following and see if you notice any shifts in your attitude and results.

★ Facing a mountain of laundry?
Be thankful that your family have decent clothes to wear.
And that washing machines were invented!

★ Yet another supermarket trip?
Appreciate the convenience of your supplies being ready and waiting.
And the good fortune that you have the money to pay for them.

★ Loathe emptying the dishwasher?
Be grateful that it's done the washing and drying for you.

★ Bored of tidying up toys?

Consider how grateful you are to have been blessed with children.

And so on...

Every thought that sets off down the road of boredom (or indeed any negative thought pattern) can be diverted via gratitude. When you first begin this practice, it will require conscious effort. But it will soon become a habit and when a sense of gratitude is ever-present and automatic, contentment and serenity will not be far behind.

Although gratitude is a great device for breaking through the domestic tedium, it will also work in any aspect of your life. It's such a powerful tool, why not enjoy the benefits of extending it beyond the home? Be thankful for everything that makes you glad! A sunrise. Your child's laughter. Your favourite TV show. Muffins. Wine. Music. Spring. Once you start - it's difficult to stop! (Proof again that what you focus on grows.) So stop looking at your ironing pile (though that will probably still grow anyway...) and cast around for the good stuff. You'll find there's plenty of it, once you start to look.

Note: An appreciation of your blessings need not be a religious endeavour. If you are of no particular faith, give thanks to the universe, or Mother Nature, or your luck or your choices. Whoever you hold responsible for the good in your life will appreciate your gratitude (even if that's you).

## The thank you effect

Whilst gratitude on a universal level can offset boredom, gratitude on a personal level can foster harmony, respect, and more importantly, help with the housework!

Time to harness the power of two little words.

How do you feel when somebody thanks you unexpectedly? How do you feel if they neglect to thank you when they should have? It's surprising the power contained in those two little words - the power to make you feel appreciated and loved...or taken for granted and ignored. For a close-to-home example, think of how you feel when someone thanks you for washing their clothes or cooking their tea. That small recognition makes you far more likely to donate your services again - even happily! That's the thank you effect.

You can use this power, not to exploit, but to *encourage* a little more help from your family members... The next time a family member does something helpful, however small, thank them. It may be a fleeting and rare occurrence, but seize it. Be visibly grateful. Shower them with praise. (Though make sure it's sincere praise - don't go overboard or it may be misinterpreted as sarcasm and backfire on you.) You may not see an immediate effect but rest assured, you are laying the foundations for future cooperativeness. An appreciated person is far more likely to want to help.

(Now you may feel this shouldn't be necessary - that they ought to help out without the gushing display. Perhaps you're right. But do you want to be right or do you want to see more of the helpfulness?)

There is a double bonus to this practice. According to the law of karma (i.e., you reap what you sow), when you are regularly appreciative of others, as if by magic, they begin to appreciate you more! So, appreciating the ones you live with will not only result in more help around the house, it will also have the happy side affect of your family finally appreciating you!

Mahatma Gandhi said, 'Be the change you want to see in the world'. In other words, lead by example. So if the idea of some recognition for all you do about the place appeals to you, why not kick-start the awesome power of 'thank you'?

You'll be grateful, I promise.

# The Heart Sinks vs The Heart Soars

Do you ever smile when you are bored? I'll venture that you don't. It's impossible to be simultaneously positive and negative. If you're feeling up, you can't be down, and vice versa.

A woeful boredom is a downer, a negative, it saps your spirit and makes your heart sink. To counteract or prevent this boredom, one thing you can do is pepper your home and your life with things that make you smile. I call these the Heart Soars. A Heart Soar is anything that makes you feel good, that lifts your spirit or your mood. We are all different, so these will vary widely from person to person. Personally, I'm a huge fan of beautiful everyday items or techno-gadgets. For example, if I must do the washing up, it adds a touch of pleasure for me to use a cool designer washing-up brush. Or if I must mop the floor, I like to have a gizmo that makes that chore easier and a tad more fun. These are small little smile-provokers that liven up essential mundane activities.

The Japanese have a similar idea behind their love of ritual. Think of the beautiful geishas in those elegant tea rooms. They turn an everyday act - pouring tea - into an exquisite performance. A joy.

Now, I'm not suggesting you adopt a kimono to go about your daily duties. But just be on the look-out for anything that could add a touch of spice to everyday domesticity. Another favourite trick of mine is to decant things into attractive jars or bottles. In my house, a vast array of breakfast cereals are virtually a permanent fixture on the kitchen worktop. The array of gaudy open packets would drive me mad. So instead I transfer the contents to glass jars and arrange them, pick-and-mix style, on a shelf - like an old-fashioned sweet shop. In this way I've turned a potential bore (constantly putting away the packets) into something that makes me think fondly of my childhood.

Now I will concede that some of these methods aren't without effort. And you may be wondering if I can seriously be advocating ideas that involve more work. But in the battle against boredom, I believe they're worth the extra labour. If the crux of the problem is not the volume of the work, but its mind-numbing nature, then it's more important to reduce your angst than your workload. Plus it's my firm belief that anything that makes you feel good is worth doing anyway.

Also, don't feel that you need to spend money to achieve these spiritual lifts. They need not be expensive items. One of my favourite objects in my kitchen is a pebble sculpture that my husband made. It makes me happy whenever I see it. Perhaps you have children who bring you 'masterpieces' or objets d'art. Any item that brings you joy will work its magic if only you'll keep them where you see them or use them.

That said, and at the risk of perpetuating a sexist stereotype, I will admit that I do also enjoy buying nice things. And I am unapologetic - what's the point of money (or life for that matter) if not to be enjoyed wherever possible. So, if and when you can, why not indulge yourself? Treat yourself to any little luxuries that warm your heart or recharge your soul.

Anything that is a Heart Soar for you will act as an antidote to boredom, so ensure you have a good collection of them within your home. They will raise your spirits and lift you above the tedium, like little rays of sunshine on otherwise cloudy days.

# Work that boredom!

An element of boredom in domestic work is inescapable. And in the spirit of going with unstoppable flows, instead of fighting this - let's see if we can use it to our advantage...

Time to view boredom in a new light.

Instead of a negative condition to be avoided at all costs, perhaps boredom can be a useful, even beneficial, state. Your chores may indeed be boring but that doesn't mean you can't get something out of them. Believe it or not, there are occasions when boring can be good.

Boredom is downtime for your brain, time off, time out. During boring activities, your brain is not being challenged or requested to work very hard. In fact, many of the yawn-inducing aspects of housework can actually be done on auto-pilot - with little or no conscious thought at all. These fallow periods can have tremendous psychological benefits but they can also be good for your physical health and your spiritual well-being.

Unchallenging repetitive movements - think wiping, sweeping, vacuuming, ironing, etc, actually lull your brain into a highly relaxed and healthful state. It's like meditation in motion. Repetitive activities trigger a relaxation mechanism which can lower blood pressure and heart-rate, promote natural healing, dissipate stress, boost creativity and improve concentration.

So those boring, monotonous tasks can actually be good for you - mind, body and soul. Just think of the potential health benefits in a house full of repetitive chores!

## Dust, vacuum...meditate.

Gentle, repetitive, rhythmical activity can produce similar effects to meditation. In both, conscious thought is radically reduced, you relax, become calm, quiet. You may be physically active, but since it is not taxing or challenging work, your mind has a chance to become still. Your chores can become a moving meditation.

But what are the advantages of this Zen nature of housework?

Eastern cultures have known the benefits of meditation since ancient times. Although it's less commonplace in the West, it is gaining in popularity. Meditative pursuits such as yoga, Zen, tai chi, etc, are becoming increasingly fashionable and mainstream. Even science is beginning to back up what our Eastern cousins have known all along. Recent research shows an improved health and well-being, even longevity, of those who regularly experience a meditative state. It appears that the mental calm and clarity of meditation brings with it a raft of favourable effects.

The benefits of regularly experiencing a meditative state include:

- ★ Increased energy
- ★ Clarity of thought
- ★ Forgiveness
- ★ Deeper levels of relaxation
- ★ Normal blood pressure
- ★ Reduced anxiety
- ★ Improved self-confidence
- ★ Increased serotonin production
- ★ Boost to immune system
- ★ Strengthening against allergies
- ★ Reduced PMS
- ★ Aid to natural healing

Research has also revealed that meditation helps to combat viruses and emotional distress, whilst boosting 'natural-killer cells', which fend off bacteria and cancer cells. All from just stilling the mind on a regular basis. So, for health and overall well-being, it seems that mind-numbing is good.

Now if only we had some mind-numbing tasks to do…

## Dust, vacuum…create.

The results of housework are all too fleeting. You spend your time performing boring tasks and before long, they need doing again. There's not much scope for any earth-shattering achievements, right?

Wrong! A surprising side effect of monotonous jobs is the activation of your creative mind. The 'mindless', 'empty-headed' state that comes from boring jobs is actually a fertile ground for creative thought, intuition, problem-solving, even flashes of genius. This productive state is known as the alpha state - which is brain-speak for a deeply relaxed mental state. It occurs during daydreaming, idle reflection, and just before and after sleep. And during housework.

Contrary to expectations, when we switch off our brains, we don't become witless zombies. We are actually primed to tap inner sources of inventiveness and imagination. According to the *New York Times*, neuroscientists have found that even when the brain is disengaged, it is still highly active. And this activity operates on a higher level to everyday thinking. This downtime for your brain actually gives you access to intelligence which is denied to the busy, conscious mind. Stilling the mind sets the mental scene for your greatest ideas!

For proof of this, think of when and where the great minds had their light-bulb moments. Archimedes was in the bath (highly relaxed) when he shouted 'Eureka!' Einstein was out walking (moving meditation) when he discovered the theory of relativity. Newton was chilling out under an apple tree (brain downtime) when the law of gravity struck him (literally!). You may even have had your own Eureka moments. Have you ever struggled with a problem or dilemma, only to have the answer 'pop into your head' when you were doing some mundane activity?

> Yet it is in our idleness, in our dreams, that the submerged truth sometimes comes to the top.
>
> Virginia Woolf

The brain is particularly receptive to inspiration and creativity during unchallenging, 'brainless' tasks - in the shower, driving, washing-up. This very book is a case in point - the idea for it occurred to me as I was on my hands and knees scrubbing the kitchen floor. And I'm in good company - Agatha Christie, a prolific imaginer, famously remarked, 'The best time to plan a book is while you are doing the dishes.'

A bored mind is also susceptible to intuition. Women are renowned for their ability to tap into this unknown element (which curiously, and wonderfully, seems to always have our best interest at heart). This may be a gender thing. But it may also be linked to the fact that women have traditionally spent the majority of their time in the home, raising children, building nests. These quiet, contemplative activities are the kind that scientists now believe connect us to some universal intelligence, aka intuition.

It would seem, then, that there is merit in boredom. It can be a prelude to creativity, problem-solving and innovation. So if boredom is a feature of your life - don't fight it! Even if you can't bring yourself to embrace it, at least turn it to good use. Though to the outside world you may look like you're just dusting and vacuuming, inside your mind, powerful forces are at work. And these forces are not only conducive to creative inspiration, they also trigger the information sorting part of the brain. So be encouraged that you're not only straightening up your house - you're performing crucial filing-work in your mind, too.

## Dust, vacuum...pray.

If you're of a religious nature, you can obliterate the boredom of housework by turning it into an act of prayer.

There is an old proverb that says, 'God is in the dishes'. This recognises a truth that many of the spiritual leaders have confirmed - your spiritual life is not only the time spent in prayer or your place of worship. Your whole life can be an act of prayer, including the mundane and the ordinary. In fact, it's possible that in these quiet, unassuming moments, we are our closest to the divine.

> Trust God.
> Clean house.
> Help others.
>
> Dr Bob
> (Alcoholics
> Anonymous)

Here are a few ways in which your domestic life can work in harmony with your spiritual path.

**Prayer.** One way to offset the boring nature of housework is to use the empty brain-space as a time for prayer. This is a surprisingly easy habit to adopt. If you have a chore that you find particularly mind-numbing, allocate that job as your prayer time. You will eventually reach a point when it becomes automatic. This trick is doubly powerful - you stop focusing on the boredom and you make room in your life for more prayer.

**Gratitude.** If you are blessed with home and family, you could offer up their maintenance as a prayer of gratitude. When you're in a spirit of thankfulness, you'll be less concerned with what housework does (or doesn't do) for you. Being grateful makes you inclined to give back. You focus less on *What's in it for me?* and think more of what you can offer in return for your blessings. You go from a place of self-centred frustration to a spirit of gratitude - which is a much more positive and enjoyable frame of mind.

**Quiet.** Places of worship tend to be hushed or silent affairs. This is because a lack of noise or stimulation is conducive to prayer. So if you find yourself home alone with a few boring, unchallenging tasks, you actually have the perfect conditions for connecting with the divine. Performing quiet activities, in a quiet place with a quiet mind - you are well-placed for the quiet whisperings of the spirit.

**Honour.** In days of old, men were driven to build elaborate cathedrals, sometimes working on creations that would not be finished in their lifetime. What force could inspire that kind of dedication? A desire to devote their life and work to the greater glory of God. Their belief was to reflect the heavenly glory in their earthly creations. It's possible to perform a similar tribute in our homes, albeit on a less grand scale. If you decide that your home can be your small way of honouring your creator, you will find more enthusiasm for its upkeep. When the work is fueled by the energy of your heart and soul, you'll find yourself less prone to thoughts of boredom.

**Peace.** According to David Carlson in *Don't Sweat the Small Stuff* (a book that changed my life), when you *allow* feelings of boredom, rather than fight them, they turn to feelings of peace. You break through the urge to entertain your mind and, with practice, are able to relax. (Imagine how lovely your home would be if housework were your chosen method of relaxation!)

**Sacrifice.** Many religions refer to the benefits of sacrifice. The idea is to undertake a loss or suffering for the good of others or to cleanse the spirit. Whilst we may no longer advocate the slaughter of the innocents, to endure unpleasant activities for the benefit of others is a form of sacrifice. To do this willingly and with an open heart will reap spiritual rewards for you as well as increase the harmony in your home. Call it sacrificial boredom.

**Giving.** In his wise and wonderful little book, *The Prophet*, Kahlil Gibran says, 'Work is love made visible.' If you have to do mind-numbing chores anyway, doing them in a spirit of giving and love for your family will have a doubly positive effect. Firstly, when you do the work in spirit of generosity, it matters less if the work is boring - the object is not to stimulate you but to offer a gift. The second benefit is in the joy to be found in the act of giving. To voluntarily devote your time and energy to others can make you feel really good. (And your soul gets a few brownie points, too!)

There are a number of books devoted to the spiritual element of the domestic regime. My current favourite is *Zen & the Art of Housekeeping*. I have also been inspired by *Prayers for the Domestic Church: A Handbook for Worship in the Home* which opens with this pearl of domestic wisdom: 'The first altar around which primitive people worshipped was the hearth, whose open-fire burned in the center of the home.'

## The ultimate in multi-tasking

As we've seen, the state of boredom can be very productive. And these benefits and activities can successfully be undertaken whilst performing all those mundane jobs. Not only that, in your bored frame of mind, you are setting the scene for some of the most transformative benefits of your life. Whilst doing the housework! Surely that is the ultimate in multi-tasking? Some people spend years on mountaintops trying to find enlightenment. Or they wrestle with creative blocks, trying to free their inner muse. Or they devote large portions of their life exclusively to prayer. Yet you can achieve some, if not all, of these effects whilst simultaneously providing yourself and your family with a pleasant environment.

And as a double bonus, these effects continue even after the work/meditation/inspiration/prayer is over. Regular periods of this quiet state can reduce stress and anxiety, improve learning, encourage better work habits and instill a spirit of cooperation. The after-effects of a little productive boredom are a calmer, smarter and friendlier you.

So the next time you find yourself in a numbed trance courtesy of your domestic routine, remember that you're achieving far more than a spot of housework. You're improving your mental, physical, emotional and spiritual health. And these benefits to your life and your health will linger (long after the visible results of your labour have been demolished by your family...).

# The power of now

From mindlessness to mindfulness. Or, how to turn boredom into enlightenment.

Mindfulness is a technique of focusing on the present, the now, the task in hand. It sounds simple enough but in practice, it can be quite difficult. Our minds are used to constantly racing ahead, wondering what we will do next. Or often, in the case of housework, what we would rather be doing instead.

Practicing mindfulness during housework is especially tricky because the mind is particularly prone to wandering during dull or repetitive tasks. A bored mind will cast around desperately to find something, anything, more interesting. In some cases it can latch onto something serene or creative - this is good. But sometimes, (you may have experienced this) the mind will hurtle off down a more negative path, such as, *This is so boring! I must get this over with. Quick, quick, quick, I want to be doing something else...!* This route is not so good.

Also, not only is frustration and resentment unpleasant, *in the moment*, but whatever we resist tends to persist. So by angrily ranting through our boring jobs, we are inadvertently setting ourselves up for more of the same. On these occasions, then, it would serve us to reign in this unsettled, restless mentality - what Buddhists call 'monkey mind'. When you experience that nagging sensation that you want to be elsewhere, when your mind is racing and your nerves are on edge - that's when the practice of mindfulness can help.

> The ability to be in the present moment is a major component of mental wellness.
>
> Abraham Maslow

The trouble is, focusing on the present moment seems to be a forgotten art. Modern life tends to drown our ability to just be, in the moment. We are bombarded with demands for our attention, constantly being beckoned to the next thing. We are in a perpetual race, rushing onward in a bid to achieve this or acquire that. We've lost the ability, even the inclination, to just stop and smell the roses.

The good news is, though, once you begin to practice mindfulness, it gets easier and easier. And the even better news is that once you can manage it, the benefits are considerable.

These include:

★ Improved performance

★ More efficiency and, as a result, speed

★ Increased powers of concentration

★ Less stress

★ More peace

In other words, you'll make a better job of it, you'll do it in the best way and in the fastest time, whilst improving your mental skills and calming your soul. You may even enjoy it! Imagine that, finding joy, peace and serenity in those mundane, monotonous jobs. You may think only Zen teachers or enlightened souls experience joy in the ordinary, but it's a trick that's open to anybody. All it takes is a little practice, and the 'mind' to do it.

> The point of power is always in the present moment.
>
> *Louise L Hay*

If you find, at first, that your mind keeps wandering, and if it's wandering to a good place - just let it. If however, you're heading rant-wards, I find the following trick to be useful in bringing my focus back to the present: I imagine I'm calmly describing the scene to an adorably curious small child. For example, *Here I am on this sunny day, running the water into the sink. The bubbles are starting to grow. Oooh, it's lovely and warm. Now I'm putting the big shiny pan in the water - soon it will be sparkling clean...* You get the idea.

Although this seems completely inane, it forces you to focus. It keeps you in the present moment. It's even more effective if you use all your senses - not just what you can see, but what sounds you can hear, or smells you can detect. What does it feel like and, if you're cooking or baking - how does it taste? This practice will train your brain to find any pleasant or enjoyable aspect in the job. It's only because we are so jaded that we fail to find any joy in our work. If some people find pleasure in domestic chores (and believe it or not, they do!), then there must be pleasure to be found. Being mindful is one way, perhaps the only way, to discover it.

## The task in hand

Boredom is relative. Often you resent a tedious task because you're focussing on what you'd rather be doing instead. What if you (temporarily) forgot about all the other stuff? If thinking about it is only causing you frustration, stop thinking about it! Just *for the moment*. Instead, accept that you are going to do the job that's before you. And once you've decided to do it, stop torturing yourself with what you're missing out on. (Also, if you keep reminding yourself how dull it is, remember - what you focus on grows...)

The challenge is in the moment, the time is always now.

*James Arthur Baldwin*

Many religions and success experts support the value of doing small things well, however mundane they appear. The idea is to commit to the job, giving it your full attention. That way, you can relax into the time it will take to complete it. You calm the frantic mind. A bonus of this approach is that you will most likely do the job more quickly. When you concentrate on a task, you become more effective, and less clumsy or accident prone. Have you ever tried to do something in such a rush that it caused accidents and ended up taking far longer than it should have? This is the principle behind the sayings: 'More haste, less speed,' and 'Haste makes waste.' Oddly, taking your time, in a focused manner makes you more efficient. So those boring jobs will get done faster - isn't that reason enough to adopt this technique?

Another advantage of being present in your work is that you will undoubtedly do a better job. There is satisfaction in a job well done which applies to any job, no matter how ordinary. It's a pride thing, an ego-boost. It may 'only' be a well-made bed or a spotless sink, but it feels good to know we have done something well. (Plus they say success breeds success, so who know where these minor accomplishments will lead...?)

## What's the rush?

What is the pace of your life? Is it a pace you are happy with? Most of us feel we are constantly rushing around trying to meet busy schedules. That's why the boring stuff bothers us so much, because there is so much else to do. But do we ever get ahead? Where does all the rushing get us? And where, dare we ask, is the finish line?

One of the most profound and helpful ideas I've ever come across was again courtesy of the brilliant Richard Carlson. In *Don't Sweat the*

*Small Stuff*, he suggests that when we die, our 'in-tray' won't be empty. In other words, we'll never get *everything* done. Never! However much you think you're ahead, there will always be more to do.

At first glance this may seem depressing, but actually it contains a wonderful enlightenment. There is peace in this realisation because it means that you can relax, *now*. This moment, or any moment. Stop trying to get everything done - because you never will. It's impossible, but also - it's not what life's about. Is the reason we're here simply to check off a lifelong 'To Do' list? I don't claim to know the answer to the eternal question of existence, but I believe we are here for the journey, not the baggage.

So why not try out a calmer, more present pace? Slow down and notice the moments. See how it feels. It may be true that you'll get less done (though, bizarrely, it may not). Either way, you will have found more joy in the experience, more pleasure in the moment. But anyway, which would you prefer - to get ten tasks out of the way in a miserable frenzy? Or to accomplish 8 things well, with serenity and joy? (Chances are the two remaining ones will wait for you...)

## Being in the moment

Your life is simply a succession of moments, one after another. Mundane or extraordinary - moments are the stuff of life. If you dismiss the boring ones as merely unpleasant pockets of dullness, to be endured or put behind you ASAP, you are actually willing your life away. We all have a finite number of moments - so don't waste them. Get the best out of every single one! Even the boring ones. And the way to make the most of every moment is to be mindful, increase your awareness, be present. Whatever you are doing, wherever you are - be there.

After all, as our modern-day sage so succinctly puts it:

> 'Breathe. Let go. And remind yourself
> that this very moment is the only one
> you know you have for sure.'
>
> *Oprah Winfrey*

So the lesson of mindfulness is this: If you have to do something anyway, commit to it and do it well and, if possible, with joy.

> **Be happy for this moment. This moment is your life.**
>
> *Omar Khayyam*

Don't rush through it, hating every second and doing a mediocre job. Give it your full attention. Find any inherent pleasure. This will result in less tension, during, and more satisfaction, afterwards. Plus doing your best in the present moment will have a profound impact on the quality of your future moments.

Taming your mind's voracious quest for stimuli and its constant searching for something else, is truly is a step forward on the road to inner peace. And you'll leave thoughts of boredom a long way behind you.

# Section 6:

# inferiority

# I'm no good at this.

Whatever our general levels of confidence and ability, we can all be subject to moments of self-doubt, low self-esteem and a suspicion that everybody else is coping better than we are.

This applies both within the home and beyond. But a sneaking sense that we aren't keeping our homes as well as others - particularly other women - is a very common complaint. So, in my bid to help you banish Housework Blues of any description, I thought it useful to address the subject of inferiority.

However, this is one of the shortest sections in the whole book for one simple reason - it's not an actual problem. I'm going to boldly declare that you are not inferior. None of us are, however much we may sometimes feel to the contrary.

To be inferior means that you are no good, or not as good as others. Yet when it comes to cooking and cleaning, it's unlikely that you're any less *able* than the next women. If you are fit and well, domestic work is within your physical capabilities. Even if you are not physically fit, it's not beyond the wit of woman to devise ways and means to get the work done. Although you may not be *currently performing* as well as others, it doesn't necessarily follow that you can't.

So *being* inferior is not the real issue here. However, *feeling* inferior can be a very real problem. To tackle this, my intention in the following pages is not to offer solutions of how to become capable - but to convince you that you already are.

## Intention and belief

*Feeling* inferior is based on belief, not fact. Yet it is a belief that will tend to 'prove' itself to you, the more strongly you believe it. Your life (and your home) will reflect not your true potential, but what you currently believe yourself to be capable of. You may argue that you feel inferior because your home is a mess, but what if your home is a mess because you feel inferior?

If you belief that you can't do it, you are unlikely to surprise yourself. Your self-esteem will affect your attitude and approach which will dictate your results. In this way, your life and your home serve as a mirror to your self-image. They back up what you believe about yourself and your domestic capabilities.

Here's a personal example. When my children were small, I used to say, *I can't possibly keep a home spotless with two small children around.* So, with this conviction, how often do you think my home was spotless? Correct - never! Yet I've been to homes that contained small children and were kept tidy and clean (and I take my hat off to those women). Obviously it could be done, but not by me - or at least not whilst I held that particular belief.

Without getting too bogged down in the effects of belief on your inner and outer worlds, let's fast forward to the happy flip-side of all this is: if you start *believing* that you are capable - you will soon become so!

Your brain is programmed to notice the results that back up your beliefs, for good or bad. So as your new mindset begins to show improving results, you'll become even more

> You may think you can do it or you may think you can't do it; either way - you'll be right.
>
> *Henry Ford*

convinced that you are, in fact, totally capable. It's an upward spiral. (You may be familiar with its evil twin - the downward spiral? But like most things in the universe, it works both ways.)

Now this may sound too easy to be true, but such is the power of a positive mental attitude. Ask any world class athlete or wealthy business tycoon. Success on the home front is achieved the same way as success in any other area - with three vital ingredients: an intention to succeed, a desire to succeed, and an absolute belief that you can and will.

The fact that you're reading this book suggests that you're intending to improve matters. And the following techniques will help you shake off those unsupportive, and quite frankly, false beliefs that it's all beyond you. Which just leaves one factor...

## Your desire for success

If you are prone to declaring your lack of abilities, it's possible that the problem is not *solely* one of misplaced feelings of inferiority. Could there also be, lurking under the surface, a secret lack of motivation?

Claiming that you can't do something is both a reason and excuse to avoid it. The idea that you're no good at the domestic stuff rather conveniently lets you off the hook to even try. So, ask yourself - is the problem that you really can't do it? Or more simply (though infinitely understandable) that you just don't want to?

Only you can answer that, but it will pay to be honest with yourself. Ask yourself if what you really want is to avoid the work, rather than conquer it. Deep down, do you truly want to be capable of the domestic stuff?

There are no right or wrong answers here - there's no point denying or trying to suppress how you really feel. But considering these questions may help you identify the true source of your struggle. If you discover that you probably are capable, yet you still aren't doing it - then the problem isn't inferiority. It's lack of desire and motivation.

But even if that's the case, don't despair - this is still an encouraging development! You've dragged the problem out into the light and discovered its true identity. Now you know what you need to work on. (And happily Section 8 is devoted just to this issue. So, if what you need is to get motivated, solutions aplenty are waiting for you there.)

However, the fact that you are reading these pages suggests that a sense of inferiority might be contributing to your woes. So there are still many benefits to be found in the following pages. It's very likely that your Housework Blues stem from a combination of 'issues', so approaching it on all fronts will give you the best chance of success.

Besides, many of the following ideas result in improvements across your whole life - not just your housework. So read on and know that whether you have a real inferiority complex or not, pretty soon your concerns about it will be a thing of the past.

# Raise the bar

Do you honestly and truly believe that your domestic duties are absolutely beyond you? If your life depended on it, could you manage it? Of course you could. Your *actual* ability is not in question. It may help to remember that, the next time you're tempted to give up with a disheartened 'I can't do it.'

You can do it.

This is an important distinction because your achievements occur in direct proportion to your expectations of yourself. I once read somewhere the suggestion that, in life (home, finances, love, etc) we tend to get more or less *what we expect*. This hit me like a thunderbolt. I instantly thought of all the people I knew (myself included) and agreed that, yes, their lives pretty much matched what I knew of their expectations. But what shocked me more was the simple but wonderful implication of this - if you want something better, just learn how to expect it!

And so began my quest of how to raise my expectations of, and for, myself. But how exactly...? Well, in my mission to adopt this strategy for my own life, I discovered the following tactics to be helpful:

★ Train your brain

★ Boost your confidence

★ Stop making excuses

★ Focus on the positive

★ Use your strengths

★ Clarify what *you* want

★ Stop worrying what other people are thinking

For the ways and means to implement these, simply read on....

# Affirm foundation

What you hear or tell yourself, with emotion or regularity, is what you become.

Think of the sports coach who constantly tells his pupil, 'You can do it! You can do it! You can do it!' How does that person feel? More importantly, how do they perform? And it won't be long before they come to believe that they actually *can* do it. Such is the power of suggestion.

Now imagine that these powerful messages are coming from inside your own head. How much more effective will they be, on your beliefs, emotions and results? For example, in *The Dynamic Laws of Prosperity*, Catherine Ponder cites a woman whose favourite phrase is: 'I am sick and tired of....x,y,z.' Is it really surprising when this woman finds herself constantly exhausted and eventually becomes physically sick?

Be aware of what you think, because that's what you will see in your life. If you keep telling yourself that you are no good, that you can't do it, before too long, you'll have plenty of evidence that you're right.

## But what if....?

What if you begin telling yourself that, actually, you *are* capable, you *can* do this, you *will* do this! It's a subtle mind shift, imperceptible to outside observers, but the change within you (and eventually around you) will be huge. Of the many success books I've read, one theme runs through all of them, without exception: the one factor that separates the successful from the unsuccessful (in any walk of life) is *attitude*. Not skill, education, beauty, strength or background, but mindset.

The most powerful influence on your circumstances is not talent or intelligence but your *approach* - and this is good news because it is entirely within your control.

You may be thinking, *Yeah...but my attitude is all wrong, I just can't get a positive attitude*, which may be true and will continue to be so as long as you keep saying it. So stop! Make a vow, this moment, make a commitment to yourself that you will keep a check on these unhelpful thoughts. Every time one pops up, stop it in its tracks, thank it for sharing - then spin it! Turn it around, put a new and improved positive slant on it. Whatever negative notion you find yourself thinking, say the opposite. And if you want to boost the effect - say it out loud!

So instead of, *I'm rubbish at this*, say, *I'm great at this!* Or, if that's too much of a leap, try a milder version such as, *I'm becoming better at this*. You may feel foolish at first and you may not be convinced...yet. So I invite you to test the power of this.

Start with a fun exercise: Spend a day where you tell yourself *repeatedly*: *I am confident and capable. I am naturally good at this. I excel at keeping my home clean and tidy. My work is effortless because I'm so efficient and organised. My home is always beautiful and I'm confident in my abilities to keep it well.* You don't need to use these exact phrases - you get the gist. Make up your own but make sure they're extremely positive, supportive and in the *present* tense.

Just for this one day, don't analyse the accuracy of these phrases. Definitely don't counter them with, *Actually, the place looks like a dump!* Then, at bedtime, review how the day went. Did you feel any different? Did you achieve anything more than usual? I'm sure you'll be pleasantly surprised by the results.

Although this fun, short-term exercise will hopefully convince you of the power of positive thinking, for affirmations to be fully effective, you have to truly believe them. Although the repetition of something over and over can eventually wear down your defences (think of advertising and propaganda), it may take longer if your inner voice is screaming *That's not true!*

> Attitude is
> a little thing
> that makes
> a big difference.
>
> *Winston Churchill*

For example, repeating daily that your home is spotless may make you want to throw up your hands and say, *Who am I kidding? The place is a mess!* Try to avoid this reaction because it only increases your self-doubt and turns your focus to the problem, rather than the solution.

One trick of over-riding this cynical inner voice is to find the smallest element of what you want to believe that *is currently true*. For example, if you feel like you are lying or deluded when you say, *My home is immaculate*, then don't say those exact words. Rephrase it until you find something you agree with. Find an alternative affirmation, along the same lines, but more accurate right now, e.g., *I love my home when it is spotless*. Your inner critic can't argue with that.

So instead of claiming, *I manage my housework with efficiency and success,* if that is clearly not the case, declare, *I am making progress towards a beautiful home.* This latter version is undeniably true *right now* - intention alone is progress, and the fact that you are reading these pages means you're intending to find a solution, so you *are* making progress.

Once you find that germ of truth, that first baby step that you can boldly claim without fear of subconscious objection - celebrate it! Focus on it and exaggerate your joy in that initial, small achievement. This alone will boost your confidence and make you more likely to believe you can reach the larger goals. You'll become more positive about your own abilities. And once these good feelings get a foothold, your achievements will snowball until a sense of inferiority will be a dim memory.

So remember that whatever you say or think regularly and *with feeling* will feature more often in your life. But positivity and enthusiasm will turbo-boost this effect. According to certain universal laws*, positivity is much more powerful than negativity. So although bad thought habits may have unhelpful results, they will take time to manifest, whereas good thought habits work fast.

> If you don't like something, change it; if you can't change it, change the way you think about it.
>
> Mary Engelbreit

If all this 'power of positive thinking' theory leaves you bewildered or sceptical, please note that a little casual digging in this area will lead to some impressive testimonials. Einstein is probably the most notable advocate, along with other great minds from history and many of the world's religions. Perhaps a more relevant champion, though, would be the wild-haired comedienne Phyllis Diller.

Diller was a housewife and mother of five before she blazed a trail for female stand-up comedy. Although one of her stage characters was a self-deprecating, inept (and slightly unhinged) housewife, she was enormously successful and frequently credits her success, in part, to one book: Claude Bristol's *The Magic of Believing.*

---

* For more in-depth information on these ideas, a couple of good places to start are: The Secret DVD/Book/Audiobook or, for a more scientific approach, www.wealthbeyondreason.com.

This book contains insights such as 'optimistic thoughts and expecting the best, inevitably form favorable circumstances' and 'your belief about yourself and your place in the world is arguably the main determinant of your success.'

I'm not the first to suggest these ideas, nor to benefit from them. My role is simply to apply the benefits of these ideas to the domestic situation. If they are universal laws, they will work anywhere - even a messy kitchen.

There's a wealth of information and inspiration on this subject, and if it piques your interest, maybe now is the time for you to explore it. (See the Resources section at www.houseworkblues.com for further material on this topic.)

But whatever you read or hear from other sources, the most convincing proof will always be your own experience. So why not give it a go? Suspend any disbelief or cynicism (where has it got you, so far?) and try a new approach. What have you got to lose?

Believe me, once you discover the power of these positive messages, there'll be no place for an inferiority complex in the new and unstoppable you!

# The Other Woman

Inferiority is relative. It needs something or someone else to be compared to.

So a sense of inferiority arises from comparing ourselves to someone else, someone supposedly superior. Why do we do that? Is it helpful? Very often it isn't, but it can be automatic and unconscious. It's a natural human tendency. Everybody does it. Whereas men tend to compare sizes (car, salary, appendage...), women tend to compare appearance - figures, clothes, and inevitably, homes.

And as a feature of the modern age, we are increasingly exposed to media standards or celebrities' homes and lifestyles. So now we also get to judge ourselves against these additional artificially high expectations of what we feel we should be doing.

It's not surprising, then, that we can sometimes believe we're falling short of 'the norm'. I know I've been guilty of proclaiming, *I'm a rubbish housewife. I'm not as good as most women.* But if we examine this common grievance, it appears that it's not only unhelpful and unnecessary, it could also be groundless.

> We're women;
> we have
> double standards
> to live up to.
>
> *From the TV show
> 'Ally McBeal'*

Firstly, how could I possibly know how good *most women* are? I have a reasonable number of female friends, but even that's a tiny sample of the current female population.

Secondly, is there really a single standard to which 'most women' conform? And who sets this arbitrary standard anyway? If there was just me on the planet, my techniques, standards, would be the norm - who's to say they're not the right ones? Besides, why does it even matter what 'most women' are doing? We're not sheep, we're individuals.

In light of all this, then, it seems obvious that one quick route out of an inferiority complex is to stop comparing our homes with other women's houses. But that can be easier said than done. So, whilst it's certainly worth remembering there is no single 'correct standard', there is another way to approach the problem.

Instead of focusing on your perceived shortcomings, turn the spotlight onto that which you believe to be better than you. It's very likely that when you start to uncover the story behind these 'superior beings', you'll discover that your lofty view of them is based on smoke and mirrors...

## Don't believe the media

Is your marriage like a movie marriage? Are your children like the perfect darlings we see on adverts? Does your hair always look like you just stepped out of the salon?

Let's face it, no one could maintain that level of perfection. Even supermodels admit they're not as perfect as their airbrushed covers and posters. Why, then, do we sometimes feel pressured to have homes that resemble a magazine spread? Even the home in the magazine doesn't look like that all of the time! It's just a snapshot, a small time frame, until life carries on, things gather and dust accumulates.

So be careful how you relate to these 'ideal' homes. Whilst it's true that interior magazines and TV shows can be an uplifting and vicarious pleasure, keep in mind that they are usually far from the norm. They are intended to be aspirational rather than realistic - to inspire you, maybe spur you to pursue the beautiful home you admire or motivate you to make the best of what you've got.

The danger comes when these artificially perfect images depress rather than enliven. So if your reaction to them is to sigh with despair, either a) remind yourself how contrived or unlikely that one shot is, or b) look at something else!

## People lie

We all have egos. We all want people to believe a certain version of us, so we gloss over the bits that don't fit the image. I'm not suggesting your friends or peers lie to you, or you to them, but we may have a 'best side' that we'd prefer the world to see, rather than the more realistic and less flattering truth.

So there may be aspects to your domestic life that you'd rather keep quiet. But do you think you're the only one? No one is perfect (which, in my view is a good thing - it would be exhausting!). What you see isn't always the whole story. So, whilst it's good to admire those who posses the qualities you'd like, don't belittle yourself in comparison to their perfection - you are only seeing the highly-polished veneer.

## It's not a level playing field

You cannot possibly know all the facts about someone else's life. Your neighbour may have a perfect home. But she may also have staff. Or an over-zealous mother-in-law. Or obsessive-compulsive disorder.

Don't waste your energy comparing yourself unfavourably to women who seem to effortlessly pull it off. Firstly, you have no idea what effort is actually going on, behind the scenes. Secondly, you are unlikely to know the full extent of any support they may have. For example, your friend may keep an immaculate home but her husband may do all the cooking or her mother may help out with childcare or any number of scenarios that give her an unfair advantage that you may not have.

It's pointless to compare results when everyone's situation is different. So, if we're not comparing like with like, why compare at all?

**Perfect home does not equal perfect life**

There are worse problems than a messy home. Those people whom you envy may be facing issues so serious they would swap lives with you in an instant. Everyone has problems, but for some these can be severe, traumatic, life-threatening and permanent.

As depressing, exhausting and frustrating as Housework Blues can be, if they are our biggest problem, that's actually something to be thankful for.

# Set your own standards (Part II)

If you're struggling in the domestic realm, it could be useful to determine whose standards you're aiming for.

Are you trying to attain levels that you are comfortable with? Or are you striving for what you perceive to be 'the norm' - whether you want that or not? If the latter is the case, it's hardly surprising that you lack the necessary conviction to manage the work involved.

For example, let's say you have a friend whose house is always spotless and pristine, with always a batch of freshly home-baked muffins to be had. She is the archetypal domestic goddess, the socially acceptable ideal. You may feel you ought to be more like her. But do you actually *want* that?

Although our social structure may imply certain levels of domestic ability, there's only one person who gets the final say on what standards are right for you - and that's you! You're not obliged to keep up with someone else's standards. You may, for example, prefer a more relaxed, 'lived-in' look. Obviously, there are certain minimums for health and safety but beyond the basic standards of care - it's your call.

> The nicest thing about standards is that there are so many of them to choose from.
>
> *Andres S. Tannenbaum*

Your life has its unique circumstances which only you know, so only you can decide on what is appropriate. Who says children must be bathed every single night? Who says we have to eat a 3-course meal at 7pm? (Diet experts frequently suggest eating little and often.)

So if you strive for certain levels of achievement, good for you, if that's what *you* want. But do it because you want to, and not because of some exhausting notion of what is 'expected'. Get familiar and comfortable with the levels that *you* are happy with - then embrace them without apology.

## But I feel guilty...

Feelings of inferiority are often accompanied by those negative nasties, guilt and shame. These feelings are understandable responses, part of the human condition. In some senses, they can even be useful - by being so unpleasant, they serve to guide us towards less shameful or guilt-inducing ways (which will usually be much better for us overall).

They are indicators. The trick is to take note of their message, so we can move on in a more positive direction.

For example, I used to feel embarrassed or ashamed if my home was a mess or not spotlessly clean. I was miserably convinced that I was falling short of some pre-set standard for all women. But this couldn't be true because I knew of women who lived, quite happily and unashamedly, in messy, imperfect houses. So after much soul-searching, I eventually discovered that I only felt guilty when I failed to reach *my own standards*.

If people called unexpectedly and there were toys scattered about the place, I didn't mind so much or worry about what they would think. This is because evidence of my children in my family home is acceptable *to me*. However, should someone discover an area where *I myself* am disappointed, that's when I would feel small and inferior.

For me, it was failing to meet *my standards* that caused the most angst.

To give you another example from my own Hall of Shame: one of my pet hates is a food-splattered microwave. I know there are more serious offenders, but it's just one of those things that makes me feel like a failure of a housewife. Trouble is, I hate cleaning the damn thing. Even though I always cover food to prevent splatters, I have yet to successfully train my family to do the same (and they clearly have the same aversion to cleaning it...) So on occasion, it will be less than spotless. But then, it's not the most visible shame-zone - and how many of your house guests use your microwave? Well, that depends if you have a friend with a baby whose milk needs warming...

> All honor's wounds are self-inflicted.
>
> *Andrew Carnegie*

Cut to the stomach-sinking moment of said friend asking, 'Can I just use your microwave?', followed by a desperate scramble (by me) to grab the bottle and furtively warm it, hoping it wouldn't smell of last night's tea. On one occasion, though, my friend got there first. I can still remember the cringing mortification I felt about my own slovenly standards.

Though I'll admit a small relief when I later saw my friend's microwave also had that 'lived-in' look. The problem isn't so much whether your guest will mind (often they won't even notice), what matters is *if you mind*. There's a saying that what you imagine other people will think (of you, your housekeeping or your home), is actually what *you* think.

It's when you fail to meet your own standards that you're more likely to feel that stinging sense of guilt about other people's opinions.

But there is a simple way to avoid all this unnecessary self-loathing. The solution is to concentrate on *meeting your own standards first*. Prioritise those jobs that make you feel confident and capable, or the ones which have the most shame-inducing consequences if neglected. Though your home may still be far from perfect, if the jobs *you* care about are done, there'll be less for you to feel shameful or guilty about.

Prioritising like this is, in itself, empowering. You are taking control. And as you simultaneously reduce or even eradicate these unpleasant negative emotions, your feelings of inferiority will naturally follow suit.

# Sound systems

Many of us will, at some point, feel inferior to women who are coping better than we are.

But note, '*coping* better than we are' does not mean '*better* than we are'. A person may be an efficient homemaker, but it does not necessarily follow that she is a better person. The difference between us and them is not ability or intelligence or innate skill. They've just got a system in place that works. And that's all *you* need.

So instead of feeling like *you* are failing, just recognize that it's your *current system* that's at fault. Don't take it personally. The state of your home is not a reflection of your capabilities - it is a reflection of your current methods and habits. There are many ways of keeping a home and if your current approach isn't successful, it doesn't mean you'll never succeed - it's just a clue that you ought to try another way.

Developing the right mental attitude is vital if you want to conquer the domestic realm. But once you have that in place, there's also much *external assistance* available, to help you become the confident and capable homemaker that you want to be. There are scores of wonderful tips and tricks and systems that can make your life easier. Other people have tried and tested techniques that make the workload simpler/possible - so why not take advantage of their experience?

> Learn from the mistakes of others. You can't live long enough to make them all yourself.
>
> *Eleanor Roosevelt*

Keeping a home is quite a challenge, but it can be unnecessarily tough if you lack the know-how to be efficient. So don't be afraid to seek help in this department - in the form of proven systems or techniques. Being more successful in the home may be as simple as stumbling across a method that really works for you.

However, it's possible that you may try a new regime and still find little or no success. Again, this is not proof that you can't do it - it just shows you haven't found the system that's *right for you*. It may well be a case of trial and error but you will get there - as long as you don't give up. Just keep in mind your ultimate goal: becoming effortlessly capable of keeping your beautiful home and family - isn't that worth a little 'homework'?

So embark upon a mission of discovery. Tap into all the expert knowledge that's readily available. The web is a great place to start, or browse your local bookshop, or even quiz your Domestic Goddess friends. Research practical systems that have helped others, try them on for size, then just keep any that fit. (My guru of choice is the irrepressible Kim Woodburn who was a professional housekeeper for many years. My favourite of her books is *The Cleaning Bible*, which is packed with valuable information. For more recommendations, see Resources at www.houseworkblues.com)

They say knowledge is power. So if you feel you're lacking - for whatever reason - you can empower yourself simply by seeking out the information you need. If you're struggling, the answer may not be working harder, but working smarter.

# Give yourself a break

You're only human. Nobody's perfect. Everyone makes mistakes.

These are well-worn clichés but the reason they're spouted so often is because they are so true. We will all lapse from our good intentions at some point. The trick is to learn from these lapses, forgive yourself, and move on.

A friend of mine once said, 'I know I'm not a bad mother because at least when I yell at my kids, I have the decency to feel guilty about it afterwards.' I thought this was a very human and positive way to deal with any shortcomings, either with children or homes or life in general. We may try and fail - but what matters most is the trying, not the failing. If the intention is there, with practice and perseverance, you can't help but improve.

> Your mistake does not define who you are... you are your possibilities.
>
> *Oprah Winfrey*

Also, take heart that, for many women, being the perfect homemaker is not an innate talent, but an acquired skill. So, don't write yourself off if you're not a born domestic goddess. You wouldn't look at a child who hadn't yet learnt to read and write her off as a non-reader. Neither are you a non-homemaker. You're just in the *pre-accomplished* phase.

When it comes to mastering any technique or skill, studies have shown that there are four stages of progress. The first stage is *unconscious incompetence*. This is where you don't even know that what you're doing isn't working. In terms of housekeeping skills, the fact that you're reading this book suggests that you have already gone beyond this first stage.

In fact, this entire book is aimed at those of us in the second stage of household management, which is: *conscious incompetence*. This is when you're aware that things aren't going as well as they could/should be. If you feel any disappointment with your current efforts, that at least shows that you are aspiring to better. This is actually a positive development and a vital step on the path to solutions. So ditch any thoughts of failure - you're actually en route to success!

The third stage, the one to aim for initially, is *conscious competence*.

This is that happy phase when you go from 'trying and failing' to 'trying and winning'. Here you know what to do to succeed and, with some effort, can manage to do it.

And when you've been doing stage 3 for a while, you'll reach the ultimate 4th stage - *unconscious competence*. This is the Holy Grail, where success is effortless and automatic, where you have it so sussed you don't even have to think about it.

So don't worry if you are struggling at the moment. In fact, you are to be congratulated on recognising your need for improvements - you're a stage 2 graduate! By reading this book, you've taken an important step in sourcing information that will help you progress to stages 3 and 4.

Admittedly, it may take some work at first - but any new skill feels arduous when you first attempt it. Just think of riding a bike or driving a car. In time, those skills became second nature. Similarly, being a competent and capable homemaker is something you can learn and eventually do without thinking.

So, go easy on yourself. You're on your way to being an effortless success within the home. Just by seeking improvements, you are making improvements. There is value in the trying - even if you don't succeed (at first). In fact, Buddhists believe that *the intention* actually matters more than the end result. So forgive any occasional lapses and refocus on where you're heading. Use mistakes as feedback for success, rather than excuses to give up.

> Our intention creates our reality.
>
> *Wayne Dyer*

Remember - you're not a failure until you admit defeat. And the fact that you're still reading suggests there's fight left in you yet!

## Be patient

By all means, believe in miracles (they do happen) but don't be downhearted if you're not successful overnight. It's taken you a lifetime to accumulate your current habits and beliefs and it's going to take a while to reprogramme them.

Just know that however small the step in the right direction - it's still progress. Small changes can make big differences, but sometimes it may take a while.

Of course, you can decide the frequency with which you implement these changes. Obviously, the more changes, the quicker the results.

Keep in mind, though, that too much too soon will only lead to burn-out or despair. So try to find a balance and a pace that not only brings you encouraging results, but that you can also sustain in the long-term. For example, dropping one bad habit or creating one new good habit every month is a manageable pace - and just imagine the positive changes over a year!

Accept that there will inevitably be dips in your enthusiasm. Peaks and troughs are not a sign of failure or inferiority - an up-and-down rhythm is the just the way of the universe. If global economies and the weather are subject to highs and lows, surely a single person can be forgiven the odd blip.

So don't fight those occasional downswings. Just accept them for what they are and ride them out. What you're striving for is a considerable challenge. Becoming effortlessly capable at keeping a beautiful home is no mean feat. So don't be surprised if you encounter a few hiccups. But keep your eye on the prize and you'll find that as you gain momentum towards your goal, the hiccups will be less frequent and less severe.

Slump?
I ain't in no slump.
I just ain't hitting.

*Yogi Berra*

Plus, when you focus with confidence and positivity on what you want to achieve, any obstacles will have less of an impact on your ability or self-esteem. Instead of taking them to heart, you'll view them simply as 'issues' to be solved. Which is all they really are.

# What am I good at?

Success is achieved,
not by eliminating our weaknesses,
but by developing our strengths.

*Marilyn vos Savant*

If you feel that you lack traditional housekeeping talents, instead of berating yourself for your failings, turn it around - what *are* you good at?

Consider your own particular strengths and skills. What are your unique talents? When do you shine? Everyone has something that they can do well. Think of those things that you've always been naturally good at. And be honest - now is not the time for modesty. It's possible to use these *natural abilities* to your advantage, but first you need to know what they are.

If you find that you're struggling to think of an area where you excel, this does not mean you're not particularly good at anything. It just means that, for whatever reasons, you're unable to recognise your own talents, but then, many of us can be blind to our own abilities.

Luckily other people can often see more clearly what we are good at. They're more objective and since they're not influenced by issues of inadequacy, they're likely to be less dismissive or bashful. So enlist your friends or family to help you. Ask them what they consider to be your strengths. (You may well be surprised and delighted by their comments.)

Also, our pleasures give us a clue to our natural tendencies. We tend to enjoy what we are good at and be good at what we enjoy. So if you're unaware of your particular skills, instead consider what you like to do.

Once you've recognised your unique gifts, you can then incorporate these into a new approach to your workload to make it more successful and less of a strain.

When we use our talents and play to our strengths, work feels easier and magically goes more smoothly. And since one big advantage of being the primary homemaker is that you get to choose how you tackle the work - you're perfectly placed to adopt a method that's in harmony with your personality. There's more than one way to clean a house, and if you get to dictate the modus operandi, why not go with the one that suits you best?

So, armed with your list of unique talents and abilities and the ways you like to work, let's explore how we can use this knowledge to make housework less of a losing battle...

The first step is to make a conscious decision to stop forcing yourself into a regime that doesn't fit. Are you battling with techniques that you believe are *the right way*, or your mother's way, or your friend's way, etc? Perhaps you've seen an 'efficiency expert' on TV and you're trying to match their system. The truth is - what works for one may not work for all. Others may swear by a technique, *which suits them*, but it may be totally wrong for the way you think, feel or like to work.

You will be much more successful if you match *your* methods to *your* natural abilities. So give yourself permission to do it your way.

> The understanding of your type can make your perceptions clearer, your judgements sounder and your life closer to your heart's desire.
>
> *Isabel Briggs Myers*

The second step is to work out how you can apply your particular abilities to help you win the domestic battle. You need to consider how to conquer your chores, your way, using your own unique skill-set. How can you apply your strengths to your workload?

For guidance or inspiration in this area, there are some good personality profilers freely available on the internet. These assess your particular traits through a series of questions, which reveal how you tend to approach your life or your work. (My favourite is the Myers-Briggs test, which was so accurate with my profile that I actually got quite emotional. It answered some long-pondered questions about why I do the things I do.)

For example, in my quest to use my strengths to solve my domestic woes, I identified my inclinations for reading, learning, analysing and problem-solving. Then I explored how to use these skills to improve my approach to housework. This involved both some inward soul-searching and some external research (both natural tendencies for me). And the result? Dozens and dozens of ideas that could make me more efficient, capable and happy with my domestic life. (My love of writing also led me to document this journey, resulting in this book.)

By harnessing my innate desire to improve and find solutions, coupled with my natural appetite for knowledge - I found solutions in my own way, that matched my particular personality. I believe this is the key for anyone to find success - identify your strengths then incorporate them in mapping out your ideal terms and conditions.

So, over to you. How can you turn your strengths to your advantage? You are the best person to determine how these will help you in a natural and harmonious way. Your new approach will be more accurate and effective if you devise it yourself. However, just to kick-start your thought process, here are a few ways in which you can use your strengths to improve your domestic lot:

Are you good at motivating people? Why not use this skill to enlist support from your family. Or perhaps you're good at planning? Why not devise a rota? These can be very powerful tools in tackling what seems like endless chores. Or maybe you like puzzles? View your domestic chaos as a puzzle that needs you to find the clues and unlock the answers. Do you like to teach? Perfect - train your children, partner or housemate.

Efficiency is intelligent laziness.

David Dunham

If your strength is earning money, do that, then pay for domestic help - that too is a solution. (And one that has my personal vote!) There are no rules that you have to physically tackle all the work yourself. Managing and delegating are all viable routes to the same outcome. If you follow your strengths and the work gets done, it doesn't matter if it's not all done by you personally. (In fact, this idea is the secret weapon of many of the world's great achievers.)

So seek solutions that match your skill-set. When you work *with* rather than *against* your strengths you will be naturally more efficient, resulting in more success and less frustration. It can also be a real boost to your self-esteem to adopt a system that works with your unique inclinations. When you do what you enjoy and excel at - with visible results - you can't help but feel good about yourself. And rightly so.

So for a healthier ego and more comfortable home, it really is worth doing the research to suss out your talents and then make use of them. After all, isn't that what they are there for?

## Explode those inferiority myths!

When it comes to your unique abilities, don't ever be tempted to think that your strengths aren't as good as someone else's. Perhaps you wish you were better at something, like your friend, mother, great aunt? Have you ever considered that they may envy what you find effortless?

For example, I used to feel inferior to a Domestic Goddess friend of mine. Her lovely home was always spotless, whereas mine was always a mess - so I would feel that she was better than me. One day, my friend called as I was merrily unblocking my sink - I had the u-bend off, the whole thing in pieces, just getting on with it. My friend was in absolute awe! She said she'd have left it for her husband, claiming she didn't have the ability or confidence to deal with it.

Vive la différence!

*French proverb*

So she wasn't superwoman after all; she was just good at one thing and I was good at something else. Which, when you think about it, is perfect. Imagine if we were all good at the same thing - who would do the other stuff?

## As a last resort...it can be taught

Although it may be true that some women are born with a natural bent for housework (and in this instance, lucky them), remember that we're not talking about being a concert pianist - we're talking about cooking and cleaning. The bulk of this work isn't intellectually taxing. Housework uses skills and techniques that can be easily learned and habits that can be easily acquired.

So if your God-given talents lie outside the domestic realm, you may have to teach yourself a few tips and tricks. But so what? Not all accomplished people are born great - some are self-taught. Maybe your strengths are seeking out knowledge, and there is plenty out there. So go with that.

If you have to teach yourself these skills, that just means you have natural abilities for something else. So once you master the domestic realm, you'll then have another string to your bow. Far from being inferior, you're becoming multi-talented!

# Inner confidence

Confidence comes from within. Nothing outside of you will make you feel more confident unless you have the mindset to match it. Not money, fame, love, success or even... a perfect home.

If you want to feel confident about your home, you have to work on how you value yourself. Taking steps to boost your confidence in other areas of your life will be reflected in your home-life and surroundings. As you rate yourself more highly, your beliefs about what you are capable of will soar. And any longed-for improvements on the domestic front won't be far behind.

Of course, it's easy to say, 'feel more confident.' It can be less easy to actually do it. So here are a few time-proven techniques to help.

**Strike a pose.** Our view of ourself is often reflected in our physiology. Think of the child in trouble, head down, shoulders hunched. Then think of the winner on the podium, chin up, shoulders back, chest out. Adjusting your posture is a perfect example of how to 'fake it till you make it'. So for an instant boost, adopt the posture of the confident person. Go on - do it now! Try it on for size. You might find it suits you.

**Fancy pants.** Wear nice underwear. This is a favourite trick of many women. Perhaps the reason it works is because it involves doing something purely for yourself (unless you have romantic intentions...) It's not about what other people might think. This suggests that you are worth bothering about, that it's worth making an effort, even if only for yourself. Imagine what that philosophy does for your self-esteem?

**Do your thing.** What do you do that makes you feel good about yourself? When you uncover the answer - do more of that! And revel in your confidence, savour the feeling, because what you focus on will become a regular feature in your life. So ensure you spend some time doing what you love and do well, to raise your energy and your spirits. In doing this, you'll get very familiar with a feeling of confidence that will boost your natural self-esteem, creating a wonderful ripple effect across every aspect of your life.

**Everyday best.** Don't keep your best clothes for a special day. Every day is special and you deserve to feel as good as is humanly possible every moment. If looking good makes you feel good, why not do it every day? Don't underestimate the power in your appearance. When you feel good about how you look, it shows. So don't keep your best clothes hidden in the wardrobe for most of the year. Experience the confidence and pleasure of being well-dressed - on a regular basis.

**Be the smartest.** Most people don't dress up just to nip to the post office, grocer, school gate, etc... So if you're all glammed up for some reason, go somewhere ordinary or mundane. You will feel like the smartest person there. Instant ego-boost!

**Keep up appearances.** Spending time on your hair and make-up can work wonders for your confidence. Just an extra five minutes pampering can make a difference to your self-image that will last all day. A favourite indulgence of mine is a pedicure, even a DIY one. Maybe it's a girl thing, but having pretty feet is good for my self-esteem - it means I'm worth the effort. Find a small thing that makes you feel good and then do it often. You're worth it! (This is not to suggest you can't leave the house without full make-up. But if your self-esteem needs a lift - presenting your best face to the world is a great start.)

**Planning.** Planning gives you confidence because it puts you in control. Instead of being buffeted about by circumstance or the whims of others, you decide the order of the day. You'll feel less like a victim and more like the pilot of your own life. Planning your day the night before is a trick of successful people the world over, and it's good advice. So start from ahead. It not only gives you confidence, but also makes life run more smoothly - which is a nice bonus!

**Beyond housework.** If housework destroys your confidence, make sure you have other things in your life, where you do achieve. If all you have is housework and you're no good at that, it can be tempting to assume that you are no good, full-stop. Yet if you are excelling at something else, you're more likely to forgive and accept any failings within the home.

**Habits.** Those 'superior' women, the ones who appear to be effortlessly capable will, either consciously or not, have formed habits that support a spotless home or perfect family. Either learn their habits or devise your own. Habits are powerful in that they look after themselves, without conscious intervention from you. So harness the power of good habits for effortless, confident ease.

**Avoid sappers.** Identify any people, experiences, occasions, even clothes that make you feel small or diminished - then avoid them! Go to any lengths possible to limit these in your life. For me, looking smart is a confidence boost, and if I feel a bit scruffy, I feel very self-conscious. It saps my confidence, so I take steps to avoid that scenario. Seek out your own personal sappers - then exterminate!

**Make lists.** Write things down. I know what you're thinking - you make a shopping list and then leave the darn thing at home. It doesn't matter - there is magic in simply writing a thing down. It re-affirms it in your mind, clarifies your intention exactly, in ink. If you simply wrote a list and never looked at it, you'd be more likely to achieve it than if you made no list at all! Try it and see. (Of course, aide-memoirs always help; a constant visual reminder further increases your chances of achieving.)

**Avoid rushing.** Treat rushing like the enemy. Rushing makes you feel inadequate because it implies that you've messed up - either you didn't allow enough time or crammed too much into the allotted time. It's exhausting, stressful and often leads to constant apologising - not the most fertile ground for confidence-building. So take steps to avoid it; any energy spent doing this will be rewarded tenfold. Be realistic about how long things take. Don't over-commit yourself. And factor in some breathing space. Besides, if you rush through your life, what are you missing? Your life!

**Be yourself.** The closer you get to your true-self - the version of you that, deep down, you want to be - the less you'll care about what other people think. This will bring you a confidence and inner calm that is absolutely unshakable.

**Cheat.** One cheat to instantly feeling more confident: just *pretend* you do. As brilliant as the mind is, it can be tricked. It often can't differentiate between pretending and reality. (For proof of this just imagine you're sucking a lemon...) So act as if you are supremely confident and accomplished. Just try it and see! I'm sure you won't be the only one in the world whose confidence is just an act - but who can tell the difference?

Section 7:

# superiority

Housework?
Moi?

Don't they know
who I think I am?

# I wasn't meant for this.

How would you feel if someone described you as 'born to do housework'?

It's probably not the most flattering compliment you'd like to receive. Despite the traditional role of the female homemaker having endured for thousands of years, in recent times, a social stigma has arisen around domestic chores. 'Housework' has become a dirty word.

In the post-feminist years, the social view of women in the home has come to be patronising at best (think of those laundry ads), or contemptuous at worst (I've heard housewives described as lazy, bored, idle, and sad - even by other women!).

Admittedly, keeping a home is not the most glamourous occupation or earth-shattering achievement, but there are many other fields of work which are equally mundane that aren't regarded quite as disparagingly. Yet the public image of the homemaker is, literally, in the toilet.

So it's perhaps unsurprising that some women (of which I'm afraid I have been one) adopt a slight superiority complex at the mere mention of housework. Though, many women would be horrified to be considered bad at housework, there are undoubtedly some women who would be equally appalled to be regarded as good at 'the domestic stuff'.

The result of social changes in the role of women has given housework and housewifery a sense of something lowly, undesirable and, dare I say it?... beneath us. After all, if we have truly entered an age where women can 'Have it all!' - who in their right minds would opt for the thankless drudgery of domestic labour?

This modern view may be understandable and/ or forgivable. But it's based on the reasoning that taking care of yourself, your home or the people you love, is an inferior activity. Yet *all* women, in fact, all able-bodied adults, have this work to do. If you are living and breathing with a roof over your head, then part of the deal is a degree of maintenance work, if only for yourself. And if the work is an unavoidable part of life, why not be good at it? Aside from the increased self-esteem that

> If the shelves
> are dusty
> and the pots
> don't shine,
> it's because
> I have better
> things to do
> with my time.
>
> *Unknown*

comes from being capable and efficient, think how much easier this essential work would be.

Regardless of this rationale, however, few self-respecting modern women I know aspire to be good housewives. And so strong are feelings on this matter that logic goes out of the (dirty) window.

> I hate the word
> . housewife;
> I don't like the word
> home-maker either.
> I want to be called
> Domestic Goddess.
>
> *Roseanne Barr*

Logically, it would be more embarrassing to admit that you *don't* keep your home clean. For example, if we applied the same argument to personal hygiene: would you recoil at being described as 'good at keeping yourself clean'? Unlikely. No one wants to be thought of as dirty, smelly or unhygienic - here it's the lack of effort which is socially unacceptable.

Yet when it comes to the home, some women will proudly claim to be terrible at housework. This suggests that being good at housework is somehow inferior - with the nonsensical assumption that women who are bad at it are superior to women who are good at it!

## Bad attitude

As illogical as all this may be, the problem is not surprising, given the way society has rounded on the domestic habits of women. There is enormous pressure on women to be so much more than 'domestic slaves'. But however excusable this superior attitude may be, it isn't helpful for a number of reasons.

Firstly, it's unlikely to win you any friends among women who don't feel that cleaning is beneath them. By staking your claim as superior, you are thus rendering them inferior. And if we are keen on equality, (and keeping our friends), that's a no-no.

Secondly, we are biologically programmed to attend to our homes and families. It may not be fashionable to admit it, but we have evolved along this line for generations. It's going to take more than a few decades of feminism to stamp out the inborn urge in many women to nurture the home environment. If you are suppressing this urge purely to keep up a facade, it will only cause you angst. It would be far healthier for you to be true to yourself.

Thirdly, wouldn't you prefer a well-kept home environment? Coming to terms with housework (even if as a necessary evil) avoids the alternative: neglect, squalor, chaos, disharmony, ill-health - clearly not the superior option. Getting past ideas that it's all beneath you is a good step towards a more enjoyable home.

## Matter of opinion

One characteristic of this problem is caring what other people think. Or more accurately, what we think other people will think. For example, if you were alone on a desert island, there would be no superiority complex regarding housework - you would do what you felt needed doing without a care for your image. (This applies to both neat-freaks and slobs and everything in between.)

However, caring about the opinion of others is a legitimate concern - we are humans with egos to consider, so it is only natural to worry about our social masks. We somehow need to resolve the tension between what needs doing and how this affects our self-image.

But if the antidote to inferiority is confidence, what is the solution to a misplaced sense of superiority? Bringing down a peg or two? A reality check? Psychoanalysis? Hopefully not. It's very likely that just considering the issue might reveal some clues as to the root causes. You might even discover that the real problem is not housework-related at all.

Either way, if you 'have issues' with domestic work, any steps you take to resolve these will undoubtedly be worth your while. The following suggestions may be firm, but I believe they are fair - and always with your best interests at heart. The ultimate aim is to help you reach a more harmonious attitude to your domestic life, which will result in more peace - within your relationships, within your home and within your heart.

So, be brave, read on. I promise to be gentle...

# Shine your light

*Is this it?*

*Is this what my life has come to?*

*I've got so much more to offer.*

Sound familiar?

If your life is consumed by housework, no wonder you feel superior - of course you have more to offer! I don't believe that any woman on the planet has nothing more to contribute than cleaning and tidying. However, that doesn't mean we should never do it. We have more to contribute than pretty nails, but that doesn't mean we should avoid manicures!

This sense that time spent on housework is a 'waste of life' seems to be most popular among women who consider themselves particularly talented or intelligent. If you bemoan the travesty of the world being denied your gifts, then you must believe that you have something of value to offer. Which is a good thing... unless this high self-esteem is met with low self-expression.

Frustration arises from not making use of your wonderful abilities. Though the resulting resentment will be aimed squarely at what you are doing instead, namely housework, that's just the symptom. The root cause is what you are achieving (or not) in the rest of your life.

> A really great talent finds its happiness in execution.
>
> *Johann Wolfgang von Goethe*

The solution to this is simple - express all those other things you have to give! Be brilliant and talented and charming and wonderful. Go out there and shine! Express yourself. Instead of lamenting what you have to offer the world - start offering it!

Doing this will take the pressure off the domestic front. Whether the work is 'beneath you' will become less of a concern. If you have an outlet for your own particular brand of genius, you'll be less likely to begrudge a little down-time to take care of you and yours.

## Yeah, but...

I expect the natural reaction to this suggestion to be: *But I don't have time to express my talents because of all the bloody housework!*

So here's my three-pronged response to that retort:

Firstly, we always make time for the things that are truly important to us. Think how you fit in organising a wedding or Christmas, a new baby, moving home, holidays, etc. These are all time-consuming activities over and above your usual routine, yet they mysteriously get squeezed into the schedule. If you want to do something enough, you can always manage to shoehorn it into your life. (I'm afraid this begs a question which might provoke some serious soul-searching: Do you want to use and express your talents enough?)

Secondly, telling yourself you don't have time makes it a reality! Try telling yourself that you *can* (and should) squeeze in some time to express yourself - and prepare to be surprised.

Thirdly, magic happens when you follow your path. When you embark on the work that only you can do, your own unique purpose, the 'forces that be' get behind you. You will be amazed at the coincidences and opportunities that will appear. One of my favourite quotes is from Napoleon Hill's classic book on success and achievement, *Think & Grow Rich*. He writes:

'The world has a habit of making room for those people who know what they want.'

So the world is ready and waiting to make room for your brilliance. Shouldn't you at least do the same?

> Whatever you're meant to do, do it now. The conditions are always impossible.
>
> *Doris Lessing*

# Extreme housework

It's an unfortunate truth that much domestic labour will be constantly unravelled before your very eyes, every time you do it.

Keeping a healthy and supportive home may be worthwhile, but the fruits of your labour will often be demolished. Repeatedly. It's understandable that anyone who is regularly immersed in housework will feel a desperate need for some kind of concrete achievement.

So perhaps a sense of being 'better than all this' is maybe just a cry for 'something *other* than all this!' (Preferably something with tangible results...)

Here's a personal example of how this idea worked in my own life. During my second baby-break, my days consisted solely of mundane, menial chores, meeting the needs of others and then cleaning up after them. Endless laundry, meals, tidying, feeding, washing. Aside from the fleeting joys of new motherhood, I was utterly miserable. I loved my family but my entire life was taken up with their maintenance (my own was bottom of the list). I felt tortured by the question: what am I achieving in life?

I began to resent many of the chores. Then I began to avoid them. I felt like the worst woman in the world - where was my homemaker instinct? My self-esteem hit an all-time low. Ironically, though, even as I was failing on the domestic front, I still believed myself to be 'above all that stuff'. So I had the double misery of not achieving my personal goals and not doing very well with the task in hand either.

Then one day, I found myself doing some boring repetitive chore and... shock horror, I didn't mind doing it! But what had changed? Had my brain finally turned to mush? Had I discovered a new love of housework?

Neither, actually. I considered this surprising development, and realising what was different, came up with a simple conclusion.

On the day in question, I had somehow managed to squeeze in some of my writing work (something I love). It hadn't been monumentally successful but to me, *it felt like an achievement*. I'd done something I viewed as meaningful and had something lasting to show for my efforts. So when I returned to my mountain of domestic chores, I did so with less resentment and bitterness about wasting my life.

It would appear then, that to combat the misery that arises from the lack of visible achievements of housework, it would help to satisfy your sense of achievement *elsewhere*.

I'm not advocating that you throw in the tea-towel and spend all your time doing something 'more worthwhile' - that would solve one problem but create others. It's the *extreme* of unfulfilling housework that can be problem, but avoiding all housework isn't the answer either. What's missing in both scenarios is balance.

When you consider it logically, it makes perfect sense. If you have a strong need to accomplish, yet you spend your days on work with few visible results - that's an imbalance. So you need to tip back the scales, by doing something that reinstates the balance, that addresses your need to achieve.

It may be my Libran sensitivities, but I believe that the simple concept of balance is the key to inner calm. Extremes of anything are rarely the best option. If your life is tipped too far in the domestic grind, you need to counter it. Introduce something from the opposite end of the scale. And this applies to any aspect of domestic work - not just lack of accomplishments.

For example, if your problem is that housework bores you, find something that really stimulates your mind. Or if it's the futility that you resent, carve out some time to pursue more meaningful activities.

Men seem to instinctively know when they ought to insist on some 'me-time'. On the other hand, women tend to be more tolerant of these harmful imbalances. This is not surprising, given that the female role has traditionally involved meeting others' needs first. But this fact doesn't eliminate our innate human need - the need for balance. Barbara De Angelis (author of the popular book *Secrets About Life Every Woman Should Know*) offers this advice: 'Women need real moments of solitude and self-reflection to balance out how much of ourselves we give away.'

So if you suspect your 'issues' may stem from an imbalance, it's clear what you need to do. When you feel angst or fury with your domestic

> You perform better when your thoughts, feelings, emotions, goals, and values are in balance.
>
> *Brian Tracy*

chores, take it as a sign to squeeze in what's missing. Become aware of the signals: frustration, irritability, impatience, resentment, lethargy - then take the necessary steps to tip back the scales.

Pursuing a better balance in your daily life will reduce much of your resentment towards housework. So you will experience more emotional stability and psychological well-being, benefitting both your health and your happiness. And as you naturally let go of the need to prove your worth by avoiding housework, your home will become a nicer place to be, too.

# Me first

At first glance, a 'me first' attitude might seem an odd suggestion in a section about superiority. People with superiority complexes aren't famous for suppressing their own requirements. However, I'm not suggesting a pecking order for what's important - you probably have strong ideas about that already. Instead, the following theory involves the *rescheduling* of what matters to you.

Simply rearranging the order in which you meet your commitments could relieve much of your frustration. If you really, adamantly, feel that housework is 'not your thing' - then why not do 'your thing' first? If your thing is to exercise - do that first. Love to read? Give yourself permission to curl up with a book. Do whatever you feel you're missing out on *before* you tackle your chores. This way, you get the miserable pining out of your system, along with any simmering resentment.

Instead of bitterly foregoing your favourite pastimes and begrudging your housework - structure your life so you get to do your me-stuff *before* the demands kick in. This may involve getting up earlier (a chosen tactic of successful and happy people the world over) or staying up late, or dropping one non-essential commitment. Get creative. Take the necessary steps to ensure there is time for you to do whatever you love to do.

If you're not convinced it's worth the effort to squeeze this stuff into your life, think back to the last time you treated yourself to some me-time - how did you feel afterwards? Angry, begrudging and brimming with rage? No, if you're like most people, you felt generous and willing to give of yourself. When you get to do what you enjoy, you naturally want to give something in return, to pay it forward - to spread the love!

> Suffocating or repressing our identities is a sure way to undermine well-being on every level.
>
> *Dr Liz Miller*

For example, you're less likely to 'have issues' cooking the dinner for your family if you've just spent a happy hour watching your favourite TV show. Or you'll feel less resentful superiority with the ironing if you got up early and spent some time on your fledgling novel, or went for a run, or a swim, or a pedicure!

Now you may say 'I don't have time' but we can always *find* time for whatever we feel is important enough. It's a question of prioritising. If being able to pursue your interests really does matter to you, why would you not make the effort to timetable them in? And if you truly want less struggle and angst around your domestic commitments, you'll find the time to do whatever it takes.

Where there's a will, there's a way.

*Proverb*

Besides - this is fun! This exercise involves making more room in your life for the stuff you enjoy! Not only that, it will also benefit those around you. Which version of you do you think your family would prefer; the silently seething martyr, bitter at her misspent life, or the one who makes sure her own needs are met and then generously meets the needs of others?

Prioritising your needs is far from a selfish endeavour - it's an investment in your health, your family harmony and your contribution to the world. What more encouragement do you need to schedule in some fun stuff? And doing it *before* the daily grind kicks in has a double benefit - you ensure there is always time, and you go on to face your work feeling more satisfied and happy with your life.

So go on - bump yourself up the list. Give your heartfelt desires the priority they deserve. After all, if you're reading a chapter on superiority, you already know, deep down, that you're worth it.

# Defining moments

If you would rather choke than describe yourself as a housewife, it's not surprising that you would take a dim, even reluctant view, of domestic work.

Perhaps, then, this superior attitude towards housework is just a problem of definition, i.e., it's not the actual work that you resent, but the worry that you will be defined by it.

Maybe you fear that if you're good at housework, people may assume that's all there is to you. Perhaps you suspect that if you're regarded as capable within the home, you'll be dismissed as the domestic-type, whose only talent is keeping a house clean and a family fed.

With the pressures on modern women to be more than 'just a housewife', these fears are understandable. But there are a number of good reasons why such hang-ups may be both misplaced and unnecessary.

Firstly, let's explode the myth that taking care of your home typecasts you as a low achiever. In reality, the opposite is very often the case. For many high achievers, a well-kept home is far from an obstacle to their success - it's a by-product of the very attitudes that help them excel in life. Being domestically accomplished simply reflects their high standards, motivation and capability, which they apply to their lives beyond the home. So the idea that good housekeeping is the reserve of the unambitious couldn't be further from the truth. More accurately, it's the standard of excellence for many of the world's most successful people.

The hugely successful motivational speaker and author of the brilliant *Secrets of the Millionaire Mind*, T Harv Eker, has a favourite saying that would explain this phenomenon: 'How you do anything is how you do *everything*.' In other words, how you approach your home is a good indicator of your approach to life - including career and personal success.

So, if what you really want is to be defined as a successful, accomplished person - your domestic schedule can be an opportunity to begin practicing those traits. Keeping a home is quite a challenge, and the skills required (perseverance, determination, patience, a good work ethic) are the same skills that can help you become whatever it is that you *do* want to be defined as. If you aspire to success and achievement, see the domestic challenge as a training ground for developing winning habits and the traits of the greats.

Now that we've established that being competent in the home need not define you as a low achiever, what about the idea that it need not define you at all? In analysing the lowly status in domestic work, are we reading too much into it? For example, my husband does housework, but he doesn't fret about being dismissed as the domestic type. To him, it's just basic life-maintenance work that needs doing. It doesn't define him.

Could it be that your resentment of being defined as something you're not, is actually frustration at not yet defining yourself as what you want to be? If so, there is good news - you can change that! Though the bad news is - *only you* can change that. In other words, it's both up to you and down to you.

So if you strongly object to the world's current definition of you, consider what label you would be happy with. Once you've uncovered the answer, ask yourself: am I taking steps to be *that*? To shake off the worry that you'll be defined by your housework - define yourself.

> If you are
> ashamed to stand
> by your colors,
> you had better
> seek another flag.
>
> *Unknown*

This may involve some soul-searching and new commitments, but it is certainly worthwhile work. In fact, it could well be the most important thing you do in your life! It will help you discover your unique path and then embark upon it. You will become the person you want to be. This is known as living 'on purpose' or 'following your bliss' and is regarded by many as the secret to a happy life.

When you're doing what you believe you are meant to do, what makes you come alive, you'll find your perspective of life in general will radically improve. And there's a very good chance it will naturally lead you to success and fulfillment. One result is certain, though - when you define yourself as you choose, being defined by housework will become a non-issue. After all, successful, accomplished women still have homes to keep - yet to them, there's no shame in doing it because they have nothing to prove.

The irrepressibly successful Kylie Minogue proudly cites cleaning her kitchen cupboards as one of her favourite stress-busters. She can admit to this without fear of being dismissed as 'merely domestic' because she has carved out her own definition in her career. Similarly, supermodel Christy Turlington admits to finding comfort and solace in tending to her home after the whirlwind of fashion shows and global travel. For these women, domestic work is not loaded with implications of underachievement. With their self-image already established, they can accept, even enjoy, the maintenance of their homes.

Bear in mind, however, that doing this work to 'define yourself' is worthwhile purely for your own peace of mind, direction and personal development. Try not to be too concerned with what the rest of the world thinks. For a start, despite all your efforts, they will interpret you as they see fit. Secondly, you are probably the only one paying much attention to the definition, anyway. We tend to fret over what others are thinking about us when, in reality, they're giving it very little thought - they're too busying worrying about what people are thinking of them!

So move above and beyond unhelpful ideas that you are being defined by housework, and take steps to create your own definition. Whether the world notices or not, you will be far more content and probably successful, too.

Then, when you're comfortable with who you are, you'll be free to take care of your home without any damage to your self-image. You'll be able to see essential everyday chores for what they are: they are not your *raison d'être*, they're just jobs that need to be done.

> Always be a first-rate version of yourself, instead of a second-rate version of somebody else.
>
> *Judy Garland*

# Smartie Pants

When I first discovered the concept of 'limiting beliefs' (i.e., the things we tell ourselves, which aren't necessarily true but are undoubtedly limiting), I scoured my thoughts for any repeat offenders. I came across this little gem:

'Intelligent, creative women are wasted on housework.'

Now, firstly, is this true? And, more importantly, is it helpful? Writing this book helped me to discover certain merits in keeping a home. (See Section 3 – *Futility*.) This would suggest that housework is not a total waste of time, regardless of ability, talent or IQ. There is value to be found in domestic work, *even if* you're capable of so much more besides.

This was a breakthrough revelation for me - that even intelligent, creative women *should* bother with housework. And once I'd arrived at this conclusion, it then occurred to me how we could (and should) use our self-professed cleverness to our advantage.

(Warning! Once you have considered the following idea, many of your excuses for avoiding housework will be rendered null and void. Proceed only if you truly do want to make peace with housework.)

Now, I would argue that all women have more to offer then basic domestic skills. However, if some of us feel we are particularly clever and talented - shouldn't we be able to put this intellect to work - to easily manage the necessary household maintenance? With such superlative minds, why don't we make use of our talents to intelligently and creatively conquer the domestic realm?

> Intelligence is the ability to avoid doing work, yet getting the work done.
>
> *Linus Torvalds*

In other words, perhaps we ought to stop using our superiority as an excuse to avoid housework - and instead use it to get the job done.

I'm afraid it's time to put your money where your mouth is. Instead of feeling that the domestic stuff is beneath you - rise to the challenge. Prove yourself to be bigger than it. So if you notice an 'issue' (a pocket of clutter/mountain of clothes/an infestation of dust bunnies) - put your self-proclaimed intelligence to work and find a solution! Devise more efficient strategies. Implement more effective routines. Or even use your genius to invent ways and means to delegate.

Instead of worrying about wasting your abilities, work out how to use them. Bring your talents to bear on the unavoidable work before you.

When you spin that old resentful gripe and turn it to your advantage, it's a far more positive proof of your ability. In fact, it's a happy win-win situation - you get to experience the satisfaction and fulfillment that comes with making use of your brilliance, and your home gets some much longed-for TLC.

So begin using your intellect as an asset, an ally in achieving, rather than an excuse to neglect. Chuck out that old, unhelpful belief and replace it with a more supportive one:

Intelligent, creative women get housework sussed.

# Go pro

This tip is aimed at women who work or have ever worked out there in the workplace. (As if the home is a place of no work! But let's not go there...)

Requisite skills for the successful homemaker are efficiency, organisation, multi-tasking, diplomacy, productivity - and, if you're smart - negotiation and delegation. So, for working women, it shouldn't be too hard to make the leap from the commercial to the domestic. If you can manage a company, office, shop, business, staff, stock, customers, numbers, paperwork, production line, website, etc, why not bring those skills home? Literally.

If your job requires any kind of time management, planning or initiative, these are all skills you can use on the domestic front to great effect. Also, routines have always had a role in domestic management (e.g., laundry day, baking day, and so on in the old stately homes), and with good reason - routine can be an effective and efficient way of getting things done. (Plus it removes the energy-sapping dilemmas of when/if to do which tasks). Equally, people skills can come in very useful in 'encouraging' your family to do their bit.

So if you are good at implementing strategies, skilled at coordinating or gifted with the gab - consider your home your new project. Treat it like you would any other enterprise: determine what's required, then use your skills to deliver.

The benefits of this approach are twofold. Firstly, you hone your professional skills by taking on such a vast and varied challenge, making you an even more formidable force in the workplace. Plus you fast-track your success on the domestic front - now that's a worthwhile promotion!

And with such effective and efficient strategies in place, your home will become less of a place of work and more of a refuge. Which is exactly what hard-working girls deserve to come back to.

# At your service

Which is better - to serve? Or be served?

The latter would probably appeal to most people and not surprisingly, egocentric beings that we are. Besides, in recent times, the gentle art of serving others has suffered something of a bad press. For example, extremes of service have acquired some very negative associations: Servitude calls to mind endless toil and unappreciated labour. Subservience suggests lack of self-respect and low self-esteem. Subordination implies frustration and oppression.

And our role as females in society has certainly brushed up against the concept. Feminism was born as a kick against the enforced mantle of women as servants to their menfolk, their children and their homes. Although many modern women have known only the freedom of recent years, for some, subjugation may be an uncomfortable memory or even a lingering reality. As a race, women have had so much servile work forced upon them, it may be difficult to view servitude as a worthwhile voluntary option.

Even aside from gender-based reactions, in our hierarchical society, the person being served is generally held to be superior to the server. So it's hardly surprising that our ego may be uncomfortable being at the service of others. Surely if we aspire to progress socially - serving others less and being served more is the most desirable option?

Perhaps not. In our haste to reject or avoid service, we might actually be doing ourselves a *disservice*.

Although an initial reaction to a call to serve might be *What's in it for me?*, if we consider service more closely, we might discover that it contains its own hidden rewards. It's possible that we may actually profit by serving others - sometimes, quite literally.

For example, there's a theory that your rewards in life are in direct proportion to the value you contribute. The more you serve others, the more you will be served. As you give, so you get. It's the principle behind the karma philosophy. In this light, then, giving or serving is good, even if only for selfish reasons!

So when it comes to the prospect of serving others, instead of asking *Why should I?*, it might actually serve *us* to recognise the inherent rewards of service.

## A route to success

If you are ambitious, if you strive to be successful - consider your heroes. Who do you admire? How did they get to the top? What was it that made them successful?

You'll most likely discover that they provided a service of some kind. Businesses become successful because of the service they offer their customers. A particular actor, author, musician, etc, will become a superstar because of the entertainment (service) he or she provides. Any scheme that makes money is meeting a requirement or providing a solution - in short, doing something for somebody else. Service.

> Nothing liberates
> our greatness like
> the desire to help,
> the desire to serve.
>
> Marianne Williamson

Seen in this light, service is a route to achievement and success. So, far from being the occupation of the lowly members of society - it's the way of the great. If you aspire to greatness, then, it would *serve you* to embrace an attitude of service.

Of course, this is not to say that being the Laundry Fairy will guarantee stellar career advancement. But if you can come to terms with the principle of service as a good thing - both for you and for others - you will drastically reduce this aspect of angst and frustration in your domestic commitments. And with a new, more positive approach with your home and family - who knows what you will achieve elsewhere?

So if you find yourself committed to a life where you are duty-bound to serve others, take heart that you are honing a skill that has made the 'greats' great. You're following in the footsteps of your heroines. And when you embrace the idea of service, carrying out the work willingly, even joyfully (it is possible!), not only will you have a more pleasant experience, with all that good karma you're stocking up - it will be more rewarding, in every sense.

## A route to happiness

It's been said that the path to finding true happiness is in the service of others. Many people choose their vocations in life based on a desire to help or serve others - think of priests, medical staff, teachers, etc - and they find great personal gratification in doing so. It would appear that serving others is a reward in itself.

On his wonderful website, zenhabits.net, Leo Babauta has this to say about his work in hospitality: 'There are those who would disparage a career path like this as demeaning and servile, yet the call to serve others is the source of my own greatest happiness.'

Many of the world's religions regard service and love as almost interchangeable, and stress the value of serving others as a vital part of their teachings. Think of Jesus washing the apostles' feet. Or Buddhist monks who dedicate their entire life to meeting the needs of others. Mahatma Gandhi claimed, 'The best way to find yourself is to lose yourself in the service of others.' It would seem that the more enlightened souls on the planet have not only found a value in servitude, but recognised it as an essential ingredient of a happy life.

Even our society is getting behind the idea of making altruistic, selfless contributions to others. Think of celebrities doing concerts or telethons to raise money for needy causes. Or the phenomenon of charity wristbands as fashion accessories. After the materialism and excesses of previous decades, our new millennium has seen more focus on doing our bit, saving the planet, caring for our fellow humans, plants and animals. The egomania of recent times didn't lead to happiness, so we're seeking a more caring and sharing mentality as a joyful way to live. Asking, not so much what others can do for us, but what we can do for others.

> To be needed is a blessing, not a curse.
>
> *Proverb*

## Make peace with servitude

In doing housework you are performing a service to the other members of your family - albeit a reluctant one, at times. But if you can get past the mental obstacle - the frustration, fury even, that you are serving others - you can start to view your obligations in a more positive light. If serving is good for *you*, just think of the potential for rewards within your own home!

So, far from seeing your domestic commitments as an oppressive regime, try seeing it as your act of devotion, your vocation, your bit. And if it's good and right that we be of service to our fellow humans - why not do it from the comfort of your own home, for the ones you love the most? It doesn't have to be all you're about but it can certainly serve as your contribution - and a significant one at that.

If you have to perform those necessary tasks anyway, doing so with a spirit of generosity rather than resentment, will benefit everybody - and no one more than you.

# The Return of the Domestic Goddess

Like inferiority, superiority is a relative matter. It needs to be compared with something else. This 'something' may be your neighbour or friend or mother. Or it may even be an unexpressed version of yourself...

Could it be that, although you feel socially obliged to act superior to housework, in truth, you actually don't mind domestic tasks, maybe even enjoy some of them?

If you emit an emphatic *Pah! As if!*, then feel free to skip this bit. This idea is for women who secretly feel at home in the domestic arena and are only battling these urges because of some media-spun image of what women should be achieving. If you're still with me, I have good news for you - times, they are a-changing.

Despite the feminist expectations of women to step away from the kitchen sink, recent years have seen a swing back to simple domestic pleasures. Pop stars have taken up gardening. Supermodels have become addicted to knitting. Crafting is now big business. Quilting bees are on the rise. There has been an explosion of TV shows focusing on the domestic agenda - cooking, decorating, even housework has been turned into entertainment (Three cheers for Kim & Aggie!) With the rise of the domestic goddess, there is no longer shame in having the time or inclination to bake a cake.

> I love knitting and sewing, and I cook and clean and everything.
>
> *Bjork*

The 1950s, the era of the original perfect housewives, is renowned for the spotless homes and impeccable children, but it also saw a disturbing rise in alcoholism and Valium use. This time around, however, domestic pursuits are more often selected than enforced. And with this vital distinction, they can be embraced as an antidote to the hectic pace of modern life.

An undoubted pioneer of this trend is Nigella Lawson. In her book, *How to be a Domestic Goddess*, she is evangelical about the joys to be found in the simple pleasures of baking. And far from being a 'brainless housewife', Nigella is a glamourous, intelligent and enormously successful writer and businesswoman - who just happens to enjoy cooking. Not only is she gloriously unapologetic about her love of kitchen life, she has built herself a fortune round it and brought pleasure to millions in the process. (She stops short, though, of describing herself as a domestic goddess - according to her brother, Nigella 'doesn't do housework.')

So this new social acceptance, even approval, may make you less bashful about any domestic inclinations. Ultimately, though, what the rest of the world thinks only counts for so much. Though we may feel pressure to match the current social ideal, the bravest (and most likely happiest) amongst us will embrace the lifestyle that is right for them - whether it is fashionable or not. The home is the one place you can indulge secret pleasures away from judgmental eyes - and if those pleasures are a good spring clean or icing cupcakes, so be it.

> What I'm doing here is seeking to offer protection from life, solely through the means of potato, butter and cream...
>
> Nigella Lawson

So, if you've been suppressing your Inner Homemaker, now is the time to set her loose. Don your pinnies and your marigolds and throw social cares to the wind.

Now, you can say it loud, 'I'm domestic and proud!'

# Section 8:

# motivation

# I don't wanna!

Motivation. Now this is the crux of the matter.

If you could, *somehow,* become motivated to do your domestic work, you would naturally stop fighting it (and where did that ever get you?). If you were sufficiently driven towards the end result, you'd do whatever was necessary - you may even do it happily! And if you felt inspired to do it, there would be fewer dilemmas, procrastinations, dark mutterings and disgruntled stompings.

If you were doing the work for *reasons that motivated you,* the work itself would bother you less.

There is magic in motivation. This is because motivation is born from a *desire* for an end result. And desire is stronger than reason and logic. When you really don't *want* to do something, all the reasoning in the world will do little to tempt you. You'll find every excuse to not do it, or if you do start - you'll stop at the first chance you get. (Sound familiar...?)

Yet, when you actually *want* to do something, or at least the result of it being done, you're so much more likely to do it. When you're motivated, you've latched onto a desire that's strong enough to get you past your objections and towards your goal.

The burning question is, though: How do we *become motivated* to do work which we view as boring, futile, unfair, repetitive, exhausting, even demeaning? How do we inspire this vital desire?

The answer is actually very simple. We speak to that very human yet very self-centred part in all of us - we focus on what's in it for us.

Though we may like to think of ourselves as generous, caring and giving creatures (which we may well be), we are also naturally self-serving. It's in our nature. We are naturally driven by what appeals to us. Even acts of selflessness are based on how they make *us* feel. Being motivated by self-interest is simply a feature of being human.

This explains why we resent the pointlessness and injustice of much domestic work - it's because we feel short-changed. And, quite understandably, if we feel we're not getting enough back, of course we won't be driven to do the work.

However, if we can spin this around, i.e., seek out *the benefits to us,* and these are strong enough, we can then use these to motivate us to do whatever is required.

So when you really have to do something you'd much rather avoid (e.g., housework) the answer is to find and focus on what you can get out of it. And if it's something rewarding and worthwhile, you're far more likely to do it, and will resent the work less when you do.

I believe this is the only difference between those natural Domestic Goddesses and those of us who hide from the washing-up. Although it's possible that the former are stronger-willed or fiercely disciplined, I think it's far more likely that they get a certain pleasure and enjoyment from their domestic work. They're tuned in to the benefits of keeping a home and so are automatically motivated to do it.

However, there is hope for the rest of us. Because even if you aren't *naturally* motivated towards domestic work, it's possible to recreate this missing motivation. And that's what this section is all about.

Simply by being open to new perspectives, insights that hold a spark of motivation, ideas that will make you see the work in a whole new, more positive light, you'll hopefully discover that there may be something in it for you, after all.

And when you recognise and *desire* the perks of doing your chores, you'll spend far less time bemoaning your lot and begrudging your work. This alone will make you more efficient (not to mention healthier and happier), resulting in you having more time to enjoy your beautiful, harmonious, supportive home and your life beyond housework. In turn, these benefits will serve to convince you further of the advantages *to you*. Thus creating a happy upward cycle of motivation towards housework! (And this is all those Domestic Goddesses have done. They're not superhuman paragons - they're just a couple of steps ahead.)

I believe the solution to that constant inner struggle (aka Housework Blues) is to uncover the inherent rewards in your domestic work. And the following pages will help you do just that. So, for now, all you have to motivate yourself to do is read on...

> Nothing is really work unless you would rather be doing something else.
>
> J M Barrie

# Ideal Home

How sweet is your home?

The fact that you're reading this book suggests that you're dissatisfied with the present state of your home or your current system (or lack of). This suggests that you believe there must be a better way. But have you ever considered, in detail, what this 'better way' would look like? Have you given any thought to what your perfect scenario would be?

If you haven't yet done this, you're missing out on a powerful motivational force - the power of goal-setting.

Imagining the ideal scenario for your home (your goal) can be a strong motivator to taking the necessary steps to get there. Giving thought to your 'dream' solution is not mere fantasy - you are sowing those vital seeds of desire in your mind. The simple act of defining what you want (as opposed to bemoaning what you don't want), is an act of focus. And when you focus, with clarity, on a desired outcome - you unleash some formidable forces within your own mind.

> The ability to set goals is a master skill of success.
>
> *Brian Tracy*

Our brains are configured to respond to a challenge. The process of defining a goal unlocks a previously dormant potential within us. It releases energy, drive, positivity and ideas. In fact our subconscious mind, when given a problem or quandary, will work day and night towards finding the solution.

This goal-seeking mechanism is not just a skill of the born go-getters. It's available to all of us - it's a function of the human mind. And all you need to do to spark the process is turn your attention to what you want to achieve.

## Three Steps to Heaven

Many, many books have been written on the best techniques for goal-setting and there are numerous different approaches. Basically, though, the essence is a simple 3-step process.

**1. Clarity.** The first and most vital step in the setting of goals is clarity - getting a clear idea or vision of what is important to you. This is a powerful process. Even if you went no further than this one step, you'd get some surprising results. This step alone will naturally stimulate your motivation. It will also lead to unpredictable developments that move you towards your goal. Any time you invest at this stage will reap dividends.

So, pause now and consider your home. Ask yourself: *What do I really want?*

Most people think they already know what they want and they probably have a vague idea. However, if I asked you to describe *precisely* what you'd like to achieve in your home - you'd probably need to think about it. So do! After all, housework offers a great opportunity for contemplation.

> Goals are not only absolutely necessary to motivate us. They are essential to really keep us alive.
>
> *Robert H. Schuller*

The trick is to be specific. Vague wishes tend to get vague results, so flesh out your fantasy. Describe your vision in detail. Do you long for a minimalist setting that's easy to maintain? Or do you dream of hiring an army of staff? Maybe your aim is simply to not live in fear of surprise visitors (wouldn't that be nice).

Simply *clarifying* what you would dearly love to achieve will be a significant stride towards it. For example, if your goal is a routine where weekends are housework-free, this awareness alone acts as a great incentive to tackle chores during the week.

You can really have fun with this step. In fact, it's all the more powerful if you do. Start small, if that feels more comfortable, but aim to build up to greater things. The only limits are your imagination, and it really pays to think big. We rarely know our true potential - so don't put the brakes on by thinking what you could *realistically* have. After all, haven't you ever done or had something you never could have expected? Isn't it possible that your future may hold more wonderful things you haven't anticipated?

As you begin to clarify your goals, it can be helpful to use your 'issues' as signposts. For once, your bugbears can be your friends! They are highlighting a desire in you that isn't being fulfilled. In other words, when you notice a problem that really gets under your skin, take this as a clue to what you need to fix.

For example, the next time you feel the urge to scream because someone has left the kitchen in a state, pause and take note of this feedback. The anger you feel is showing you (quite strongly!) that what you desire is for your family to clean up after themselves. Congratulations, you've just clarified a goal! Although you may find that little comfort as you set about dealing with the mess, you've initiated the success-seeking guidance system in your brain. If you're open to the ideas that follow, the solution of training your family may be closer (and easier) than you ever thought possible.

**2. Write it down.** Once you've got a clear idea of your goal, write it down. Advocates of list-making will tell you there is magic in the written word - even if you never look at it again. This is because the process of writing forces you to crystallise your ideas. However, there is definitely merit in revisiting your written goals. They are a great tool in charting your progress and a useful visual reminder that reinforces your aims.

If you're in any doubt of the power of written goals, I suggest you read Mark McCormack's book, *What They Don't Teach You At Harvard Business School.* In it, he quotes some compelling statistics from a decade-long study of Harvard MBA graduates. For example, in 1979, 3% of the participating graduates had written down their goals and made plans to achieve them, 13% had unwritten goals, and the rest had no specific goals.

> People with goals succeed because they know where they're going.
>
> *Earl Nightingale*

When the graduates were interviewed 10 years later, those who had unwritten goals were earning, on average, twice as much as the graduates with no clear goals. However, the 3% who wrote down their goals were earning, on average, *ten times* as much as all the other graduates put together!

So write down your goals! Wherever this secret power comes from - make use of it. In fact authors Tom & Penelope Pauley (of richdreams.com) believe that writing it down is all you have to do! In their book, *I'm Rich Beyond My Wildest dreams, I am, I am, I am*, their suggested route to riches is simply making detailed lists of what you want. It's a fascinating and fun technique and one that I've already had some success with.

Now, you may need an open mind for this and a little faith, at first. But it's not necessary to explain or understand the forces at work to make use of this trick. Once you try it and see the evidence that it works, you'll be convinced. In fact, you'll probably be so excited and amazed that you'll want to share it with everyone! So, get yourself a nice pen, and maybe a smart new notebook in honour of your new regime, then grab a cuppa and a seat - and write down the blueprint for your perfect home-life. Then prepare to be amazed.

(Note: If you're like most people, you will now be nodding and thinking, *Yeah, yeah, I get the idea, I don't really need to actually do it...* If that's the case - reread the statistics above! This stuff works - why not make use of it to help you? It's a small effort that will reap dividends - *but only if you do it!*)

It's worth noting here that it's not necessary to know the exact route to your desired outcome. To paraphrase Martin Luther King, you don't have to see the whole staircase to take the first step. There is a school of thought that believes the answers will find you. Personally, I've had much experience of this method and find that in the act of setting a goal, a few ideas 'magically' crop up. I've learned to trust these nudgings and take inspired action.

> Leap and the net will appear.
>
> *Julia Cameron*

There may be times where I can't see how these actions could possibly result in my goal, but invariably, by some route I could never have imagined, they do.

So my personal belief is that the route will occur to you once you make the decision to go for it. If you have faith in the process, you only have to know what you want to achieve and the answers will appear as you go along. For me, this path is not only successful, but hugely enjoyable and full of magic and awe.

It's possible, though, that a more structured technique will appeal to you. If you find it helpful to map out a series of steps that could get you to your goal, that might be the best process for you. Many success experts recommend this. In *The Success Principles*, the hugely successful Jack Canfield has dedicated a chapter to this idea of 'chunking down'.

To do this, take your end-goal and reduce it down to all the steps you believe you'll need to take to get there. Make these smaller and smaller chunks until you find one you can start with.

Which brings me nicely onto the final step...

**3. Take action.** Make a start. Take the first step.

When you have outlined your goal and/or how to starting bringing it into reality, you will naturally *want* to start pursuing it. You'll have discovered that Holy Grail - motivation - which will help to drive you towards your ideal home, *as long as you take action.*

Now this may sound like the hard part - you actually have to put some effort towards your goal. But think about it, all this means is that you take steps in the direction of what you really want. Why wouldn't you want to go there?

No doubt you already expend much time, energy, even blood, sweat and tears in your domestic struggle. And where is it getting you? Why not put the same energy into a more focused programme and start seeing some of the results you crave? Instead of viewing goal-work as extra work, see it as *more efficient work*, which will actually get you closer to where you want to be.

In the book/movie, *The Secret*, Rhonda Byrne talks about a book which changed her life and brought her everything she ever dreamed of. That book was Wallace D Wattle's *The Science of Getting Rich*. In it he writes, 'Hold with faith and purpose the vision of yourself in the better environment but *act upon your present environment* with all your heart and with all your strength and with all your mind.'

> By thought,
> the thing you want
> is brought to you.
> By action you
> receive it.
>
> *Wallace D Wattles*

This is sound advice. In fact, it's the secret of success which has been passed down through the ages and used by some of the greatest people in history. Yet the very same process can be applied to the more mundane business of housework. So why not make use of it? If you truly would prefer your ideal vision of home and family life - begin taking steps towards it. Today.

## Goals and housework

If you're serious about becoming more successful on the home front (not to mention making essential work easier), goal-setting is a powerful tool. But, not only will it help you become more effective, this practice can also improve your health and your emotional well-being.

Humans are naturally goal-striving beings. Our natural state - when we are healthiest and happiest - involves working towards whatever brings us joy. So, not only do we possess these awesome abilities to achieve our goals, we actually get a kick out of the process!

When our goals are set *by us*, based on our deepest desires, we are naturally motivated towards them. We don't need persuading to take the necessary steps. We eagerly, even cheerfully, take on the work required. Even if the work is arduous (or monotonous and mind-numbing...) we're less likely to begrudge it, if we can keep our eye on the ultimate prize - a prize that is meaningful to us.

> To achieve happiness, we should make certain that we are never without an important goal.
>
> *Earl Nightingale*

In this way, you can use your desire for a calm and comfortable home to unleash the time, energy and drive to do whatever it takes - even housework. So if your goal is to get on top of your cleaning, there is comfort in the knowledge that your constant efforts are not wasted - they are moving you towards your goal. For example, you are less likely to mind tidying up a messy living room (again), if your self-certified mission is to always have somewhere comfortable and pleasant to sit and relax.

A personal goal of mine is to make sure my family are well-dressed. I get much pleasure from seeing my children in adorable clothes or my husband looking dapper. And I love the confidence boost I get from being well turned-out myself. These goals are what keep my chin up as I face all the laundering and ironing and sorting that's a necessary part of a well-presented family. Driven by the end result, I cope more positively with the action it takes to get there.

This technique of setting your goals and then focussing on the final reward, rather than the obstacles, will be triply effective. Firstly, since you can't focus on the positive and negative at the same time, you'll spend more time thinking about what you do want and less time feeling frustrated or despairing about your problems. Secondly, since what you focus on expands, you'll see more of whatever you're aiming for, whether that's a clean house, tidy living room, helpful children or cooperative spouse. Finally, setting and achieving goals is an enjoyable way to live. It's fun and rewarding to regularly get what you want. So you actually score three goals. It's a house-keeping hat trick!

To hell with circumstances; I create opportunities.

*Bruce Lee*

Part of the magic of this process comes from being *pro-active*. This sense of taking the reins in your own life ought not to be underestimated. Feelings of frustration - in life, not just the home - often arise from a sense that we're not in control of our circumstances. We fall into a pattern of just reacting to one crisis after another. Or we just drift along with whatever life throws at us - even if the current is going in the wrong direction. But once you decide to have some say in the situation, when you set an intention for specific improvements, you take back some control.

It's worth bearing in mind, however, that you may need patience. When you begin to harness the power of this technique, you will regularly achieve what you set out to do, but some larger goals may take time. So, to keep up your sense of accomplishment, it makes sense to have a number of goals of varying degrees of difficulty.

For example, an ultimate goal may be to have a pristine walk-in wardrobe, where all your beautifully laundered clothes await you. If this is important enough to you, you have the potential to achieve this. But it's unlikely to magically appear overnight. So why not set an interim goal of simply making a dent in this week's ironing pile? As you take action on your short-term goal, you're taking a small but certain step in the direction of your ideal.

So give both your large and small goals some thought. In fact, give them lots of thought. After all, how will you ever get to where you want to be, if you don't know where that is? It would be like setting out on a journey with no end-point in mind. So give your goal-seeking mechanism a head start and at least input the destination! You may or may not be aware of every stop on the journey, but with your guidance system set on the target, you will eventually get there.

Once you master this skill and experience the magic of it, you may want to use it in other areas of your life. And you should! The process works universally, not just in your home. From relationships to weight loss, wherever you would like to see more success - set a goal. And if this technique really piques your interest, you should definitely explore it further. (Brian Tracy is my goal-guru of choice and his books or audios are a great place to start.)

So, become goal-oriented. Because once you know what you're aiming for and have a mindset to achieve it, there will be no stopping you. Then, when you look around your beautiful domain and you know that you've achieved your domestic goals, ask yourself, *What do I want to conquer next?* Then go for it!

With this little pearl of goal-setting wisdom, the world truly is your oyster.

# Celebrate your triumphs

Success is naturally motivating.

'Success breeds success' may be a well-worn cliché, but it's a scientifically-proven phenomenon. It's backed up by results from neuroscience, NLP, metaphysics, even spiritualism.

The essential theory behind this is: Whatever you give your attention to, whatever you think about most of the time, will show up in your life. And the more frequently you think about it, the sooner it will appear. Plus, if you focus on it with passion, you turbo-charge the process.

This explains how successful people, who focus *with enthusiasm* on being more successful...become even more successful! Success naturally boosts positivity, confidence and optimistic expectations - which results in more successful outcomes. It's a virtuous cycle.

Now, there are many, many brilliant books, websites, seminars that go into this is much more detail and it's a fascinating, even magical, theory. (If you're keen to study it in more depth, Jack Canfield, Bob Doyle and Rhonda Byrne have some great books on the subject.) However, it's a simple idea to grasp. In, fact, you've no doubt already experienced it in your own life. Ever had a day that started badly and went downhill from there? This is the same theory - but in reverse. When you focus on what's going wrong, it affects your attitude, changes your mindset to a more negative and pessimistic outlook. This affects the decisions you make - usually with undesirable results.

In short, your thoughts affect your attitude which influences your decisions which dictate your results. Also known as: your life.

The life you have today is a result of all the previous, minute decisions that you have made up to this point. And these decisions were driven by your attitude, mindset and approach.

For example, if you hadn't still been angry about burning the toast, you might not have exploded at your child's accidental spill and you wouldn't now be feeling guilty about it (which may incur some other undesirable consequence). It's all linked. What happens in your world is a reflection of what's going on inside your head. So you can see that what you think about and focus on has a direct impact on your external reality.

If you accept this (and it is cited by many as a Universal Law, as constant and irrefutable as the Law of Gravity) you can use it to your advantage. How? By choosing to focus on the good stuff!

By all means acknowledge anything that isn't' working, *but don't dwell on it.* Use it as a springboard to find the solution. That's where your attention should be: the solution. Train yourself to recognise an 'issue' then turn all your thought and energy toward solving it. The process of focussing builds momentum - so make sure you're pointing in the right direction before it gets going!

This simple mental shift is a huge step towards your ideal situation. It's an imperceptible change of focus but it will be enormously effective in taking you closer to where you want to be.

Then, when you find and create those successful solutions (which you will, if you put your mind to it) - dwell on them! Celebrate your successes, however small. Revel in them! Give yourself a mental pat on the back. Not only is this great for your self-esteem - you are literally hardwiring your brain for bigger and better future successes.

When you celebrate a triumph, large or small, you're programming your mind to notice more of the same. You're forging stronger connections in your brain that lead to more feelings of success. You're encouraging a mindset that will notice more of your personal achievements - those wonderful things you do and forget to give yourself credit for. And the more you take conscious note of what you're doing well, the more occasions you'll find yourself doing things well. This is human psychology - it's how our brains work.

> Attitude determines altitude.
>
> *Anonymous*

You may say, *But I'm not doing anything right. I'm doing it all wrong!* (Hopefully you can now spot the consequences of even thinking along those lines.) Admittedly, it's difficult, at first, to find something to feel positive about. But even in a run of bad days, one was probably worse than the rest - so equally one was the *least* worst. Focus on what you did differently that day.

Seize upon *anything* you've done right or you'd like to see more of. Tell yourself - repeatedly - that you are capable of success in the home. You *can* get things done. You *do* achieve certain goals. Also, tell yourself that you are getting better all the time. As long as you have the intention to improve, this is never a lie.

So, become achievement-focussed. Monitor your successes. For example, if you walk in the kitchen and you see clean and clear surfaces, pause, notice and smile! This is a good thing. This is what you want to see more of. If you are responsible for it, congratulate yourself. Enjoy the feeling of accomplishment - you did that!

Aside from any metaphysical results of attracting more achievements, success itself is a great motivator. Everybody loves to feel successful. You enjoy the feeling and it encourages you to take the necessary steps to feel it again.

For a personal example, I used to feel like a failure every time I went to bed and found it still unmade. This went on for *years!* Then I decided I would become a 'bed-maker'. At first it was hard to be disciplined but what motivated me the most was the feeling of success I felt, whenever I noticed my well-made bed. Now, when I walk past the bedroom, it makes me happy to see that my bed is made. This minor triumph reminds me that, when I put my mind to it, I can turn failure into success. (By the way, I am now so naturally motivated to make my bed that most days it 'mysteriously' gets done without me even noticing I'm doing it! How's that for brain-training?)

> To succeed, we must first believe that we can.
>
> *Michael Korda*

This success principle is generally taught to people looking for business excellence or life mastery, but it applies just as much in the home. So why not make use of it? Once you understand and apply this technique - proficiency on the domestic front will naturally follow.

So go now and seek out your triumphs - large or small. Determine for yourself what makes *you* feel successful. It's your home, your life, and you know best what you'd like more of. The only rule is that you notice your successes, daily, and give them unbounded praise and credit.

Then just watch them grow.

# Wanted! Reward.

Whether we're conscious of it or not, we are driven by our desires, wants and wishes.

It may simply be a need for love, approval or recognition. But most, if not all, of our daily decisions are influenced by whatever is in it for us. This is not a consciously selfish thing, it's just how we're built, to go after the things that are important to us - otherwise, why would we have such urges?

The trouble with housework (or at least, one of the many) is that often we can't see the reward. There's no obvious payoff. You may have instinctively drawn this conclusion already, if you've ever faced your domestic chores with a despairing, *What's the point?* Although the other ideas in this book will hopefully enlighten you towards previously unseen returns (e.g., harmony, health, etc), there may be occasions when you need a little more enticing...

With this in mind, what could be more rewarding than an actual reward?

The next time you're faced with a dull task that has no visible offer of reward - create your own! Offer yourself a reward. Decide what you feel you'd deserve for doing a specific spell of domestic duties, then when you've done your bit - relax and enjoy your prize!

Not only will you then be able to revel in your absolute worthiness of it, you'll do so surrounded by less housework. But more importantly, the anticipation of your reward will spur you through the jobs, often in a fraction of the time and maybe even with a smile on your face.

The dangling carrot principle is one that works the whole world over. To get anybody to do anything, you have to offer an incentive - from children with sticker charts, to nations with trade agreements. Without this vital ingredient, all inclination may be lost, however obliged you are.

For example, you may know very well that *you ought to* do some housework, but if you can see no light at the end of the grimy tunnel, it's no wonder you can't get motivated. So create your own light!

Of course, everybody's rewards will be different. In this game, you get to choose the prize. It may be something as simple as a new magazine, a phone call to a friend, or double chocolate chip muffin.

(My self-administered reward for a spotless kitchen is a tea and cake break.) Whatever brings you a little pocket of pleasure in return for your labours is a fair trade.

Now you may be thinking, *I could just indulge in my reward without doing the work.* And you could - but how would that help you? You'd have to try and enjoy it in the still messy house, trying to ignore all the work still to be done. Plus, it would be far less satisfying. Sometimes, the rewards of labour are all the sweeter because of the work you had to do to get them.

> The reward of a thing well done is to have done it.
>
> *Ralph Waldo Emerson*

So the next time you're dwelling on how unpromising your work is, take matters into your own hands. You deserve something for your efforts and if nobody else is offering it, go and get it for yourself. And when you do, enjoy it. You've earned it.

# For the good of your health

What's the big deal about cleanliness?

If our homes are our own, to enjoy as we want, why must we all conform to the same standards of good housekeeping?

One word: health. Good hygiene is the basis of a healthful environment. Without it, it won't be long before illness becomes a regular houseguest. A neglected home can affect both your mental and physical health. It can become a breeding ground for all kinds of bugs and beasties and negative energy that rob you of your natural well-being. Some can even be fatal.

## The Microscopic Menace

I once watched a video of a bowl of rice which had been left out overnight. To the naked eye, nothing much seemed to be happening. However, with a special camera that showed the reproduction of bacteria, it made stomach-churning viewing. Before I saw that footage, I'm ashamed to say, I had quite a lax approach to putting food away. Since then, however, I don't need any encouragement to take the necessary steps to keep my food, and home, as sanitary as possible.

When we understand *why* we need to do a certain task, i.e., the consequences for us, we are far more inclined to do it. Understanding the purpose and benefits of regular dusting, vacuuming, laundering, etc may provide the prompt you need to tackle those chores. Being aware of good, even vital reasons, why housework needs doing will automatically motivate you to do it.

So here are a few details of what (or rather who) may be lurking in your home if you don't...

* ★ Dust contains allergens from house dust-mites, pet hairs and mould spores.

* ★ Up to 100,000 dust mites can live on one gram of dust.

* ★ Dust mites feast on dead skin flakes.

* ★ The average mattress holds a million dust mites, each one producing up to 20 droppings a day.

* ★ More than 60% of allergic asthma cases are caused by dust mite faeces.

★ Moulds can produces millions of airborne spores a day. These can be highly allergenic or even toxic.

★ Symptoms of dust mite allergies include: coughing, sneezing, itchy eyes, runny eyes and nose, sinus headaches, swollen sinuses, and difficulty breathing.

★ Damp leads to mould and mildew which produce toxic airborne spores.

★ In the US, food poisoning causes about 76,000,000 illnesses a year. And 5,000 deaths.

★ The common cold virus can survive on a contaminated surface for up to 18 hours.

Now, some of these facts may make you squirm, but my intention is not to make you uncomfortable in your home. On the contrary, the point is to promote a healthier home. These uninvited guests will occur whether you're aware of them or not. So by being informed, you're more likely to take steps to eradicate them. (In fact, researching and writing this section inspired me to begin my spring cleaning! How's that for motivation?)

In learning these hazards, you may even uncover the source of an existing health problem. But the main aim is to highlight the issues - and the potential harm - so you will give priority to the essential cleaning tasks in your home. Then you can relax, safe in the knowledge that your home is supportive to your health and well-being, rather than a breeding ground for allergens and toxins.

In the hope that I've done such a good job in motivating you that you want to rush off immediately and eradicate these nasties, here are a few quick tips on dealing with them:

> Our house is clean
> enough to
> be healthy,
> and dirty enough
> to be happy.
>
> *Unknown*

★ Dust mites reproduce rapidly in their ideal conditions of heat and damp. You can reduce the warmth and humidity in your home by turning down the central heating, regularly airing your rooms and soft furnishings, or using a dehumidifier.

★ Vacuuming is a more effective way of eliminating dust, as dusting can just redistribute it.

* Washing bedding at high temperatures kills dust mites.

* Putting soft toys in the freezer for a couple of days kills any inhabitants.

* Dust mites can't thrive in sunlight, so air your laundry outside when possible.

* Destroy mould with bleach or white vinegar.

Having highlighted the dangers, I feel it's only right to offer these basic solutions, but a more thorough education is beyond the scope of this book. (My job is simply to get you to *want* to seek out this information.) There are many great books available which cover effective cleaning tips and techniques in much more detail. My favourites are *Zen-cleansing*, *Home Hints & Tips* and Kim and Aggie's wonderful *Cleaning Bible*, but a few minutes on the web will also provide you with a wealth of cleaning know-how (and know-why). Then, armed with this information, you'll have a convincing incentive to take on your housework: it is, literally, for the good of your health.

(Be warned, though, once you start digging on this information - it will become harder for you to ignore your housework!)

## For sanity's sake

In your mission to enjoy your home, health ought to be your number one priority. In fact, I believe, *in life*, health ought to be your number one priority. Whatever else you achieve or accomplish, it will be a shallow victory if you lack the health to enjoy it. But just physical health is not enough. To truly appreciate and enjoy your home (and life), you need to be mentally healthful too.

In much the same way as you promote physical health through good diet and exercise, so your mental well-being needs nurturing with regular doses of R&R. And where is the place you recharge your mental batteries? For most of us, it is our home.

> He is the happiest, be he king or peasant, who finds peace in his home
>
> Johann Wolfgang von Goethe

For this reason alone, the effort you make towards a comfortable and pleasant environment will reward you with psychological balance.

This idea is a valuable and powerful motivator, so to really get the point home, I'll say it again: *the effort you make towards a comfortable and pleasant environment will reward you with psychological balance.*

It can be a great encouragement to know that, in exchange for your labour, you get a soothing refuge from the world - which is a vital ingredient for a healthful mental state. However, your domestic input will actually be doubly rewarded. This is because housekeeping has (ironically enough) been cited as a very effective antidote to depression! According to a study published in the *British Journal of Sports Medicine*, 20 minutes a day of rigorous housework can actually *improve* your mental health.

You may balk at this, claiming your chores are what cause your woes in the first place - and I know where you're coming from! But housework is a valid form of exercise and any physical exercise is beneficial to your mental health.

Also, aside from the proven medical effects of a calm home and a calm mind, it can be gently cathartic to bring order from chaos. There is something mentally soothing about transforming grubby and grimy into spotless and bright. So, cleaning and tidying can offer psychological boosts in their own right.

> It's all in the attitude - housework is exercise. Slim your way to a clean home!
>
> *Linda Solegato*

Note, however, that you will only receive these inherent benefits *if you are open to them.* You'll need to suspend any anger or frustration when you tackle your chores and open your heart and mind to the simple joys of domestic tasks. (No, I haven't lost the plot - these do exist! Ask Martha Stewart.)

When you stop resisting and resenting the work (and where did that ever get you?), you may discover that the work can actually *lift* your spirits, rather than dampen them. So, if you have to do the work anyway, stop fighting it! By approaching your workload with a positive frame of mind, not only will you boost your mental health, you'll also have a much more enjoyable experience.

And once you've made peace with this essential maintenance work, you'll feel less inclined to avoid it. You'll take back control of your home and in doing so, you'll bypass that downward spiral of overwhelm and fury which can so often lead to despair.

So try to view at least some of your housework as a worthwhile investment in your mental health. Keep in mind that you're safeguarding your sanity and setting the scene for increased serenity and calm - which will, in turn, leave you better placed (and more likely) to tackle the work involved. It's a positive and healthful win-win.

A robust and happy state of mind is priceless, yet a degree of effort on the home front more than fits the bill.

# The first 1% is the hardest...

According to Mark Twain, the secret to getting ahead is getting started.

He makes it sound so easy. But the reason it is such a powerful move is because often it's the most difficult one. So how do we motivate ourselves to tackle our chores when just beginning is such an overwhelming obstacle? Well, here's a little tactic that just might do the trick...

Ask yourself - what is the absolute bare minimum you could do, to qualify as 'started'? Then just do that one thing!

Forget about the entire job - you'll never make it that far if you don't conquer the beginning of it. Initially, just focus on the tricky business of making a start.

To help you discover what the first step will be, you could pretend your most prized possession depended on starting the job. What would be the very first thing you would do? Then, once you know - just do that.

Or you could pretend your job description is Designated Starter. For example, if the prospect of dealing with a sink full of pots is just too much to bear, try pretending that you're part of a team, and your only responsibility is to kick-off the job. So, what do you need to do? Empty the sink? Run some water? Find the easiest, most basic task that will fulfill the requirement of 'making a start'.

Once you reduce a heart-sinking chore to its first baby-step - you are so much more likely to begin it. And beyond that step, it will be less of a mental barrier. You've pushed past your resistance and suddenly, it doesn't appear quite so daunting. Then, with the most difficult part behind you, it can only get easier.

It's surprising how much of a psychological barrier *beginning* can be. And knowing that getting started is the most difficult part can be a good motivator to just get that bit done, to just get started, if nothing else, to get the greatest hurdle behind you.

As Confucius eloquently remarked, 'The journey of a thousand miles begins with a single step.' Or, perhaps less profoundly but equally practical, Mary Poppins put it this way: 'A job begun is half done.'

So get into the habit of 'just beginning'. It's a skill that will improve the more you do it - what better excuse to *make a start?*

# ...& the last 1% is tough, too.

What's the difference between finished and almost finished?

Surely it's just a case of tying up a few last loose ends? After all, the majority of the work has been done. And our natural tendency is to slacken off towards the end of a task, making the final stages particularly tough. So, is it really worth forcing ourselves to push through to completion?

YES! It is! Resisting the temptation to fall at the final hurdle brings *massive benefits*.

This is because our brains love a sense of completion. Although, logically, the difference between 99% and 100% is only a fraction, the psychological effect from that final 1% is huge. In fact, our brains get so much pleasure from the conclusion of a task, that they reward us, literally, with a surge of happy-hormones!

According to Brian Tracy, author of *Goals*, when you complete a task of any kind, your brain releases a small quantity of endorphins. He says, 'This natural morphine, Nature's Wonder Drug, gives you a sense of well-being and elation. It makes you feel happy and peaceful. It stimulates your creativity and improves your personality.' That's quite a rush! All from that final 1%.

> There are two kinds of people, those who finish what they start and so on...
>
> *Robert Byrne*

This process works whatever the size of the task. Admittedly, the more important the challenge, the greater the endorphin-rush on completion, but even the fulfillment of small tasks can make you feel happy and exhilarated.

Knowing that you'll experience this thrill can provide some much needed motivation to get you through the final stages. But perhaps even more compelling is the lasting effect these mini-successes will have on your self-esteem and self-image. The positive results of these minor triumphs go way beyond the task in hand.

Developing an attitude of achievement *in anything* improves your chances of success every aspect of your life. When you regularly *feel* like you're winning, (even if it's only against the Laundry Mountain!), it won't be too long before you *become* a winner - in whatever you set your mind to.

An entire philosophy of success (Psycho-Cybernetics) is built on this idea. Studies on the human brain have shown that creating and focusing on small successes in everyday life is the basis for more monumental success in any area you choose - health, wealth, career.

When you experience that winning feeling, your internal machinery is set for success.

*Maxwell Maltz*

When you know, with confidence, that you habitually complete whatever you set out to do, you become unstoppable. So whatever your ambitions beyond the home, you can greatly improve your chances of achieving them, simply by finishing those seemingly unimportant domestic chores.

In addition to helping you achieve more, there are emotional benefits to totally completing your tasks. For proof of this, picture the reverse. How do you feel about unfinished tasks? Those niggling little jobs are so-called for a reason. The dictionary defines 'niggle' as: a slight but persistent annoyance, discomfort or anxiety. That last 1% may be proportionately small - but it can really bug you!

Incomplete actions are a major source of stress and anxiety. They rob you of mental and emotional energy, affecting your mood and very often your sleep. Compare this to the feeling of elation and relief when you complete the task, and you wonder, *why didn't I do it sooner and save all that stress and worry?*

So, it's in your own interests to aim for 100% completion. The only trouble is... it's very tempting (and common) to ease off towards the end of a task, to stop when you are 'more or less' finished. Total completion will not usually be the easiest option (in the short term). At times, it may take Herculean efforts to get there.

But completing is a skill and like any skill, when practiced, it gets easier. The more you force yourself to finish tasks, the more automatic it will become. You'll develop a completion-habit. You'll become a natural finisher.

It may also help to keep in mind the triple whammy of benefits that come from completing a task. Firstly, there's the enjoyable (not to mention healthful) physical high from the endorphin rush. Secondly, you experience a heightened sense of achievement and capability -

with long-lasting and powerfully positive results. And thirdly, you reduce a good deal of unnecessary angst and stress from your life.

Being aware of these benefits can be very motivating. So when you're tempted to give up at 'almost done', just keep in mind that winning feeling. Remember that by resisting the temptation to give up, you're embedding a powerful message in your self-image. You are training yourself to become someone who gets things done. Simply anticipating the good feelings and the boost to your self-esteem can give you the extra drive you need to finish that final 1%.

So, recognise that you'll naturally resist those final efforts, but you can fight this temptation by keeping your eye on the prizes of completion. You can discipline yourself to power through to the finish line. Though these last efforts may feel like the toughest, they will be the most rewarding. They carry with them the promise of satisfaction, fulfillment and a mind set for success.

And this positive mental attitude is the Holy Grail, for greater accomplishment and achievement within the home, and beyond.

# Home vs career?

How can you possibly advance up the ladder of success, if your time and talents are spent chipping dried Cheerios off the kitchen table?

I have often posed this question to myself (and anyone else unfortunate enough to be within earshot). On those days when all I've done is clean and tidy my home, I've found myself thinking - is this really all I'm good for? What about my ambitions? How can I be a success in life with all this housework to do?

> I think housework is the reason most women go to the office.
>
> *Heloise Cruse*

If you're even remotely ambitious, yet have some domestic duties, you can probably relate. It's easy to view any housework as the antithesis of career success. But, in recent years, I have learned that the two need not be mutually exclusive. In fact, I've actually come to believe that they may be intrinsically linked...

Firstly, there's the obvious connection highlighted in the practice of feng shui. Eastern cultures have long believed in a correlation between the state of the career section of your home (the North) and your success in the workplace. In feng shui terms, clutter and grime are bad chi (energy) which can negatively influence your life, even beyond the home. Luckily, though, the reverse is true. Encouraging good, healthy chi in your home (i.e., keeping it clean and tidy), can actively energise all areas of your life - including your career.

Renowned feng shui expert, Lillian Too, states, 'Good feng shui expands your career, presents opportunities for promotion and helps to attract mentors and other patrons who can improve your prospects.'

So, if you yearn for fame and fortune, you could do worse then have a tidy up in your Northern sector. But then, why stop there? Your health and relationships can also impact your career success, so you could well benefit from ensuring these areas (East) are well-kept too. If you'd also like to add financial success to the mix, you'll need to spruce up your Southeast sectors. And if your ambition is to marry well, get scrubbing in your Southwest quarters!

If you are open to these ideas, they can serve as powerful motivation to keep on top of your domestic chores. When knowing you *ought to* do the work is not enough to get you through it, picturing the advantages of good chi can be a much more effective incentive.

On a personal note, I've noticed over the years that whenever I have a big sort-out or a good spring clean, it acts like a magnet to 'Lady Luck'. Good things seem to happen. I don't claim to know how this works exactly, but I've learned to just go with it. After all, I don't need to understand combustion theory to enjoy the benefits of my car. So, in blissful ignorance of *how* tidying my office results in an unexpected windfall - I just get on with enjoying my new-found cash!

Sandy Forster (International Mentor of the Year 2008) offers this explanation on her website wildlywealthy.com: 'The Universe abhors a vacuum. Create a space for your prosperity and it will be filled. Get rid of the clutter in your life – the books you don't read, the paperwork in your drawers, the old clothes that don't fit, the boxes of junk in the garage. When you clean out the old, you make room for the new – so start creating that space for abundance today.'

It's true that the direct connection between housework and a blossoming career may not always be clear - in fact you may never know which results arose from your domestic efforts. But in opting to keep your home well, you're erring on the side of success. If there are invisible forces at work - wouldn't you rather have them working in your favour?

> Make room for the things you have worked for, prayed for and so strongly desire.
>
> *Catherine Ponder*

So, if you set any store by the power of unseen energies, you'll give your career a considerable boost by making peace with your domestic demons. But feng shui advocates are not the only ones to suggest that your housekeeping habits can impact your lot in life. In her book, *Women & Money*, finance expert Suze Orman is emphatic about the link between a tidy, orderly home and the state of your finances. According to her, good housekeeping is not just a precursor to career success - but a prerequisite.

This makes sense. A supportive home is like a foundation that equips you to cope with the rest of your life. When your foundation is strong, you are able to achieve greater things than if you come from a base of chaos and ill-health. So maybe there is some truth in the adage of 'cluttered home, cluttered mind'.

Organisation, good systems, efficient strategies, these are all the hallmarks of successful people, who apply these skills, not just in business, but in life. When was the last time you entered the office or home of a person who was at the top of their field and found the surfaces covered in clutter? Mess and success aren't natural bedfellows in the workplace. It appears the same may be true within the home.

For proof of this, think of the effect your home has on your mood, your energy and your self-esteem. Then consider how these factors affect your career performance. Put this way, the link between the state of your home and your aspirations seems obvious. And in recognising this link, you begin to see *real advantages* in taking care of your home. If you are at all success-focused, this can be hugely motivating with regard to housework. If you have big career dreams and ambitions, this insight can help you to see housework, not as an obstacle to your advancement, but as *an integral part of your success*.

Also, bear in mind that having the time to take care of your home does not mean you have failed in life. In fact, with the modern pursuit of work-life balance, the freedom to enjoy simple domestic pleasures is fast becoming a barometer for true success. Gone are the days when furs and fast cars were the ultimate goal. Now it seems that an abundance of *time* to spend on home and family is the achievement of choice. Success is becoming more about lifestyle than status symbols.

> An unhurried sense of time is in itself a form of wealth.
>
> *Bonnie Friedman*

Hopefully this will help you get past the idea that domestic work is subordinate to *real* work. The two can, and do, complement each other. So not only does your home play an important role in your success, having the time to give it the love and attention it deserves is, in itself, a considerable achievement.

However career-focussed you are, there will always be some housekeeping to be done, even if it's just tidying up before the cleaner arrives. And by embracing the idea that home-care can work in harmony with your ambitions, you'll be infinitely happier as you are doing it.

# Get ahead. Stay ahead.

Getting ahead is a reward in itself.

There is much satisfaction to be found in being ahead of the game. It feels good to think you are competent, on top of things, in control. And once you discover this great feeling, it can be a strong motivation to do future jobs before they become urgent.

I learned this one the hard way...

For many years, I hated the morning rush. I'd drag myself out of bed at the last possible moment, then panic as I tried to iron the required uniforms and feed and dress the children in time to beat the school bell. Tense, rushing, and stressed, I would have a very short fuse. My poor offspring would often trudge to the school door with some angry reprimand ringing in their ears. Obviously not the best start to their day, or mine.

Then, one Sunday evening, I called a friend and she mentioned that she'd just finished ironing the uniforms for the week. It was like a Eureka moment! I drifted off to a wistful vision of clean pressed uniforms, hanging, waiting in the wardrobe, one for every day of the coming week. It seemed like a dream compared to my temper-torn scenario. Yet all it would take was a little planning and about half-an-hour of scheduled ironing...

> One who does not look ahead remains behind.
>
> *Brazilian Proverb*

And so it became my weekend routine. In fact, it feels not just sensible but somehow right, a relaxed wind-down from the weekend, ready for a new week. And once I coordinated it with a favourite Sunday night TV show, the habit was set. So now, even though school mornings can still be a little hectic, it's in a lively, bustling sense. (Rather than a growl-at-any-passing-child way - which is certainly an improvement.)

So I use the promise of calmer school mornings to inspire me to do the work *ahead of time*. In fact, I have since become such a convert to the perks of planning and anticipating any potential flash-points, that I apply this technique to many other areas of my life. I find that by dealing with things in advance, life seems to just flow so much more smoothly. There are real joys and advantages in getting ahead. And knowing this gives me that essential motivation to get ahead.

However, you'll only ever be totally convinced by this phenomenon when you experience it for yourself. So I invite you to try it. Cast your mind over your commitments, particularly the ones that leave you frazzled or stressed. Then look for ways in which you could get ahead of the game.

Discipline weighs ounces, regret weighs tons.

*Jim Rohn*

Initially, you might struggle to motivate yourself to put in any effort before it becomes a screaming deadline. If so, just try picturing how it would be if you did get ahead, imagine how much more pleasant the situation could be. Visualising in this way can serve as a good interim motivator. However, the real magic will come once you get a taste of being on top. It's a feeling you'll want to repeat. The more you experience the sense of being serenely in control, the more you'll be motivated to take steps to be there again in the future.

## Peak performance

Now, let's fast-forward to that happy day where you've managed to get your home back on track and you're regularly ahead of the game. The good news is, you've made it - you're on top. However, the bad news is... you're not finished yet.

Almost as tricky as *getting* on top of your domestic commitments, is *staying* on top.

Allow me to give you an example of how easy it would be to start heading back down the slippery slope to chaos. Picture the scene: You've just finished tidying, you're all done, so you move on to something else. Then you see a wayward sock out of the corner of your eye. Just one sock, not doing much harm. It hardly renders the place an utter pigsty. Surely it can wait till the next tidy up...

Wrong! If your aim is to hold on to that winning feeling of being in control, you're going to need bulletproof self-discipline. It may be only one sock but it is also the seed of mess, clutter and chaos. If you let this one go, it will multiply while you're not watching. The next time you see it, it'll have been joined by its old friends the Empty Cup and the Abandoned Toy. Before you know it, the room will be categorised as a mess and will make you want to collapse in despair, that ahead-of-the-game-feeling a distant memory.

You need to nip these offending mess-magnets in the bud. To avoid the rapid downward spiral, you'll need to pounce at the first intruder, no matter how seemingly innocent or insignificant. Be spurred on by the knowledge that if you let this slide, all your hard work in striving to the top will have been in vain.

Plus, if you're motivated by the thought of an easy life, remember that it's usually easier to deal with jobs immediately. For example, if you come across a solitary pot in an otherwise spotless kitchen, it's not a mammoth task to dispatch it back to its cupboard. If there's just a single item that needs attention, you're more likely to deal with it straightaway. However, if you see several cups, a few plates, glasses, cereal-caked bowls and maybe a pan or two... you'll probably want to just leave the room. You are far less inclined towards a bigger effort. So remember - a small job, when left, will grow! Making the decision to deal with small job *now* avoids having to face a big job later. So tackle the little blighters whilst they're young!

Keeping this in mind will be a great incentive to deal with offending items as soon as you spot them. If you've managed to claw your way to the top (and I take my hat of to you), do whatever it takes to stay there. It is so much easier to *keep* a place clean and tidy, than to *get* a place clean and tidy. It's like scaling a mountain. How satisfying and easy is it to be at the top - compared to the struggle of the climb? So if you've done the hard bit, stick your flag in the ground and stake your claim. Defend your territory against any marauding socks, mugs, toys or other invading detritus.

As an added incentive, once you're committed on this route, you'll unleash the awesome power of habit-forming. When you repeatedly deal with each job immediately, without question, that wee small voice that likes to procrastinate will soon get fed up of you consistently ignoring it. Eventually it will stop objecting and before you know it, you'll be dealing with the vast majority of your domestic chores *without even realising it!* Surely that's the ideal way to cope with the daily grind? All those chores that used to irritate and frustrate you, will be magically completed on auto-pilot.

> Motivation is what gets you started.
> Habit is what keeps you going.
>
> Jim Rohn

You'll have reached the dizzy heights of the Automatic Domestic Goddess, where getting ahead - and staying there - will be a breeze.

# Start the clock

There is a school of good housekeeping that suggests you use a timer in your daily routine. The idea is that you allocate a certain amount of time to a task or room, then you get on with it until the timer rings. You decide in advance how much time you're prepared to devote to your chores and then you do just that, and no more.

I can see the merits of this system - it prevents the energy-sapping notion that you're spending your whole life doing housework. And if you work well within a rigid structure, you may find that it suits you to run your home, literally, like clockwork. If this does appeal to you, then the fly lady website (www.flylady.net) is an inspiring resource.

Personally, though, this system is not for me. I'm not a huge fan of deadlines, particularly self-imposed ones. I believe there's enough external pressure in my life, without introducing a ringing bell into my housework.

However, there is one aspect of this system that I find very useful. One helpful side effect of timing your chores is that you get a more realistic idea of how long they *actually* take, i.e., in reality, rather than *in your head*.

I believe that often we feel so resistant to a job that it builds up in our minds. We erect a psychological barrier to it, out of all proportion to the work involved. The thought of it becomes a much bigger deal than the actual job itself.

For example, I recall a time shortly after the birth of my second child when I left the washing-up for three days! (I know, I know...) My mother came round and I moaned for a couple of hours about how I was just drowning in housework. My wonderful mum listened and sympathised. Then, while I nipped off to change a nappy, she washed up. It took her about 10 minutes.

My point is that if I had been thinking in terms of how long it would take, I'm sure I could have found 10 minutes, in preference to the angst of having it sitting there, staring at me, getting me down. But I was more focused on my frustration and failings. I let that particular source of despair loom large as a giant chore in my mind. It wasn't a giant chore. It was 10 minutes work. (It might even have taken less than 10 minutes if I'd dealt with it sooner...)

The lesson I learned was this: When I feel any resistance towards a certain job, I consider how long it will realistically take. I can then weigh up that time against the emotional angst I will subject myself to, if I *don't* do it.

It makes sense. If you have to do the work anyway, tackling it early on could save you much heartache. And one very effective way to motivate yourself to do this, is to reduce it down to $x$ minutes work.

And if you aren't already familiar with how long it takes to do your chores, there's only one way to find out! I don't suggest you go as far as setting a timer - unless you find that a positive encouragement. A casual glance at the clock as you start and finish a particular job is all that's needed. But as you time yourself, go at the pace you like to work. It's no good setting the world record for cleaning the loo, then being disappointed the next time when it takes you twice as long.

So, check the time, go as fast as you comfortably can whilst still doing a good job, then log that time in your mind. You can then use that knowledge in future, when you're wondering if you have time to do that particular job.

For example, I used to have issues with emptying the dishwasher. I would put it off all day, as the awaiting dirty pots would stack up around the kitchen. Then one day I clocked how long it actually took to do it - about 2 or 3 minutes! I was letting a couple of minutes-worth of work rob me of a tidy kitchen for the whole day. When you view it like that, it looks insane! So I acquired the habit of doing it as I wait for the kettle to boil for my morning cuppa. That is truly all it takes, then it's done.

Timing your jobs can be an eye-opening exercise. You discover those jobs that have been niggling you for days can be dispatched in a matter of moments. And you feel so much better in the process!

> One must learn a different sense of time, one that depends more on small amounts than big ones.
>
> *Sister Mary Paul*

In fact, you may be surprised by how much satisfaction you can get from such tiny spells of effort. In the same way that the idea of a job grows out of all proportion if you *don't* do it, when you actually take it on, the sense of competence and efficiency is exponential. Jobs that would have bugged you all day are suddenly behind you, leaving you feeling supremely capable and adept.

The mere act of analysing the timescale moves you from a place of despair and overwhelm into a much more positive mindset. It forces you to focus on the solution rather than the problem, which is the key to success in any activity.

So instead of walking into a messy kitchen and dwelling on the heart-sinking feeling, look past the (negative) emotion to the bare facts, i.e., there's about 15 minutes work to do. This approach will help you get the job done so much more quickly and effectively. Plus it makes you far more likely to tackle the work at all.

Another advantage of knowing how long jobs *really* take is that you are more likely to (voluntarily) deal with them in idle moments. For example, if you have a spare five minutes before you have to leave, instead of killing that time, you might use it to put a laundry load in. Or as you're waiting for the toaster, you might empty the kitchen bin.

Don't underestimate the effect of a few minutes work, here and there. This is the way you will reclaim your home - and your life. After all, your workload built up gradually overtime, and that is the best, most sustainable way to retaliate - little and often.

So the next time you see a job that you've been avoiding, ask yourself: how long will it *really* take? The little voice in your head may claim that you don't have time to do it now, but you can more easily quieten that voice if you know it's only a 1 or 2 minute job. Then before you know it, it will be done. You can then go about the rest of your day feeling less oppressed by what needs doing. In return for a few moments' effort, you have lightened your load a little.

When you begin to see the magic in these small moments, you'll be far more inclined to tackle the miniature battles. And this minute-by-minute approach will lead you to greater victory in the domestic realm.

# Fix your toolkit

Want to make your workload easier? Less time-consuming? More enjoyable?

There is one simple step you can take which simultaneously lighten your existing load and make you more inclined to meet your domestic challenges. What could this doubly effective strategy possibly be?

Simply recognising the value of a decent toolkit.

Any task will be made significantly easier, more efficient and enjoyable when you have the right tools for the job. So consider your current domestic toolkit - are you armed with the best tools available to you? If not, why not? Using inadequate, inefficient tools is causing you *unnecessary* struggle. Haven't you got enough to do without making your workload more arduous or time-consuming than it needs to be?

Fixing your toolkit is one way of working smarter, not harder.

So give high priority to any devices or technology that makes your life easier. Decent tools have real value. If you dismiss the importance of these, or struggle to justify the expense, just be aware that coping without them also incurs a cost. The cost is in the way you spend your time. You are spending your precious life-moments on these tasks. So, in short, you are paying with the quality of your life.

Admittedly, there may an up-front investment. You may have to spend some time researching the best equipment, but this will reap dividends. If you read reviews (the internet is great for this) or talk to your friends, you are likely to avoid costly mistakes. You can also invest a little more time in tracking down the best price. By doing this, you can get even more quality for your money. And when you know the best products and where to buy them - buy the best you can afford. Quality may cost you more but you have to decide what is your ultimate goal? To have an enjoyable, supportive home and an easier time caring for it? Or more money in the bank.

> The quality of life is more important than life itself.
>
> Nobel Prize winner
> Alexis Carrel

When weighing up how much you are prepared to pay, consider the true cost of not buying the best you can afford. Seething your way through the weekly ironing pile with a decrepit iron will have a cost on the quality of your life whilst you're doing that work (which will take you longer...) Not to mention the adverse affect that simmering resentment can have on both your health, your relationships and your looks. So you may end up with unnecessary furrows on more than just your clothes! Bearing in mind the cost of anti-wrinkle creams, does the cost of a new iron seem like a better investment?

So do whatever is in your power to ease your workload. With a little forethought and investment in a decent toolkit, not only will you spend less of your life on your jobs (can you think of a better incentive?), you will also be less frustrated and resentful when you are doing them. When you have adequate, quality, even pleasant tools, the job is instantly easier. And when your jobs are less of a struggle, you are more inclined to do them.

This way, domestic success lies.

Note: You needn't draw the line at mere efficiency. Add anything to your toolkit that makes you smile. If leopard-print rubber gloves tickle your fancy - go for it! If you prefer to wipe sparkly granite worktops, good for you! Whatever gives your domestic life a boost of pleasure is worth its weight in gold.

If you are going to spend a significant portion of your life doing this work, paying for the resources that make it easier or more pleasurable will be money well spent. They're not a frivolous extravagance - they're an investment in the enjoyment of your home and your life.

And who can put a price on that?

# Let me entertain you!

'People are coming!'

In my house, this is the one occasion when housework gets priority. There's no time for philosophical musings over the futility and injustice. My pride is at stake. It's a code red - panic cleaning.

I think it's pretty safe to say that most of us care what other people think of our home. However much we claim otherwise, our egos like to keep up appearances. No matter how comfortable we are with our 'relaxed' standards in the privacy of our own home, having them made public is another matter.

Nobody wants to be thought of as a lazy slob.

This may be vanity (or, in some cases, fraud) but it's just human nature. We all have our social masks - which are usually a more flattering and respectable version of ourselves.

However, it would be exhausting to maintain these appearances, to be permanently on show. So it's only to be expected that we let the image slip at home, away from the gaze of the world. Even the Victorians had less-than-perfect private quarters, where a guest would never be admitted. But for those of us who don't have the option of dedicated receiving rooms, what happens when we allow the public spotlight into our private refuge? What do we do when (eek!) we're expecting company?

We unleash the surprising power of House Pride. This substantial source of energy, which can lay dormant until threatened with impending visitors, can be stirred up and used as a force for good.

> Mummy, why are you cleaning? Is somebody coming?
>
> *Joshua Raine*
> *(my son)*

When you are expecting guests, you magically find the motivation to get the housework done. Jobs that you haven't bothered to do for your own enjoyment, you will do for your guest's approval. Or rather, you will do to keep up a certain image. We want to maintain the facade - however removed it is from the truth, however bulging the out-of-bounds cupboards where you shoved everything.

Pride is a great motivator.

So, if you really want to conquer your domestic work, yet can't find a convincing incentive - invite people round! If you need the prospect of company to make your home presentable, plan for that. Exploit the fact that the idea of guests turns you into a whirlwind of domestic accomplishments.

At first glance, you may think this proposal is insane. When you don't want to do housework - why would you voluntarily *invite* pressure that will force you to do housework? But the truth is, sometimes, we indulge in self-sabotaging behaviour. Though, deep down, we want a clean and tidy home, we 'inexplicably' avoid the cleaning and tidying!

So it may be time for a self-administered kick in the rear, to make us do what it takes to get what we really want (in this case, a clean and tidy home). Without the threat of visitors, you may make (and accept) excuses to not do the work. Whereas putting your public image on the line is a surefire way to get you going.

Arranging for guests to come will hopefully inspire a zero-tolerance approach to mess and grime. The pressure will lift your game, ensure that you perform.

In fact, I know of some women who use a version of this trick but without the live guests. They *pretend* they have friends arriving and spruce up the place accordingly. Whilst I applaud their discipline and imagination, I personally need the very real prospect of approaching guests to motivate me. Otherwise, I may pretend that my imaginary guest probably won't need to use the loo, so won't bother cleaning it. Whereas (after many previous, cringing experiences), I'm well aware that real guests will *always* need to use the facilities - *especially* when you haven't cleaned them!

So, if your ultimate goal is a pleasant and comfortable home environment, and you truly long to find the motivation - this is an ego-powered solution. Picturing how proud and competent you will feel as you welcome you're guests into your beautiful home is a powerful driving force. The desire for that feeling will help you find the energy to roll up your sleeves and go for it.

A happy side effect of this may be a boost to your social calendar! When you invite people into your (beautiful) home, you will often get a return invitation to theirs. So you get a nice evening out in reward for your efforts. (More than likely, they will also have the pre-guest frenzy in anticipation of your arrival and approval!)

But the main reward will be the home you get to relax in when your house-guests have gone. You may be quite surprised at the joy and satisfaction you feel as you look around your newly gorgeous domain. (I have been known to take photos of it looking that good, since I know it will be fleeting...)

In all likelihood, you'll find yourself thinking, *My home looks so fabulous! Why don't I always keep it like this?* And your brief glimpse into this well-kept new world may just inspire you to stay there.

# The 'Joy' of Mealtimes

'What's for tea?'

How do you feel when you hear this? There are days in my house when all I can offer in response is a doleful sigh. Surely they don't need feeding *again*? But they do and they will.

When you think about it, the frequency and variety of meals required by most households is considerable. Now wonder it can leave even the keenest cooks feeling a little jaded. Although cooking can be a joy, being responsible for the provision of a constant and endless stream of meals can become a strain. Especially if you have to pander to the whims of fussy eaters, preparing numerous bespoke platters at every mealtime.

As a child my family's menu consisted of two choices: take it or leave it.

*Buddy Hackett*

Of course there are easy options and cheats - which I believe have a helpful place - but these can't be a daily solution. If you are the primary cook, your family's health and well-being are in your hands. So, this is one aspect of your schedule that is worth doing well.

With this in mind, it pays to face up to this culinary challenge, to come to terms with exactly with is required. And in my quest to do precisely that, I've uncovered a few helpful tactics that will enlighten and motivate you kitchen-wards. And armed with this new mindset, you may come to find a certain competence and satisfaction, maybe even joy, in your provision of meals for others.

So, pull up a chair and dig in. It's chow time!

## Plan, Shop, Chop

I was once reading a cookbook by that original domestic goddess, Nigella Lawson. In it, she casually mentioned that planning and shopping are as much a part of cooking as the kitchen-based business. This was a lightbulb moment for me. Of course! It seemed so obvious when pointed out! Yet all this time I'd been wondering why I felt so defeated by the prospect of feeding my family. I had neglected to incorporate two of the three vital ingredients - planning and shopping.

I recalled that, often it wasn't the prospect of *making* the tea that made me want to hide in a darkened room, it was the effort of *thinking* what on earth I could cook. And how I expected to feed a family without a little prior grocery shopping, I don't know.

Success in any venture is much easier when you know what's required before you start. So, if you are struggling on the culinary front - it will help you to consider the *prep work* of the process. If you can acquire the habit of planning ahead - it will make your kitchen-life much less of a battlezone.

And if you still need a little prompting in this department - focus on the potential for pleasure. This is *shopping* we're talking about! If you have a tendency towards retail therapy - here's a chance for a guilt-free spree. And shop where you actually enjoy the experience. If you're going to spend a good proportion of your time restocking supplies, you may as well eke out any gratification to be had. Go to your favourite supermarket, or market or deli. The advantage of it being down to you is that you can do it your way.

You're going to have to face 'What's for dinner?' at some point. And you're going to need the wherewithal to make it. Giving some thought to these aspects earlier, rather than later, not only makes for better meals, it also makes for an easier life *for you*.

Now isn't that more to your taste?

## Build a Repertoire

This is a very simple but effective strategy. Although technically, it's a practical hint, there will be benefits to your confidence and self-esteem. And when you believe you can easily cope, you tend to do just that.

*Write down* your kitchen repertoire. We all have a certain meal we can make without consulting a cook book, possibly without even thinking. This information is already in your head, but putting it on paper clarifies it. It makes you more aware. Plus, it will also provide you with a written reminder of what you're capable of, on those days when you simply cannot think what to cook.

You may also be surprised at how accomplished you already are. Once you begin your list, you'll start remembering all those meals you can make with your eyes closed. You may even be inspired to add new dishes to your list. And if you were to learn just one new recipe a month, for example, your repertoire will soon be pretty impressive.

Knowing you have an armoury of meals that you can make easily and without too much thought will be some comfort when you are next called upon to do so. (Which probably won't be far off...)

## Pick up a cook book

This tip really works for me. I find that when I browse a really nice cook book - it makes me *want* to cook. It provokes some kind of innate desire in me to provide delicious, nutritious meals for my loved ones. How's that for motivation?

The key to this, however, is timing. If you grab the book minutes before the children's tea-time (or worse, before hungry guests are due) the pressure will kill the experience. But if you do this in a quiet moment, *in advance*, without any expectation or panicked cries of *What on earth can I cook?*, you may be surprised...

As you casually peruse lovely pictures of scrumptious food, you just might be inspired. You may see something that catches your eye, something you actually *want* to make. Many modern cookbooks are objects of beauty in their own right, with beautiful photography or design. So just relax, enjoy it and be open to ideas.

If a certain picture looks appealing, or a certain recipe sounds delicious, go with it. Make a mental note of the ingredients or stick them on your shopping list. (I have been known to be so inspired by a recipe that I immediately ventured out to track down the ingredients.) Even if nothing strikes you immediately, on a sub-conscious level, you are reinforcing food and cooking as something pleasurable, rather than just another chore.

> Cooking is like love. It should be entered into with abandon or not at all.
>
> *Harriet van Horne*

So if your cooking has lost its flavour, dig out your cook books! If you don't have any, visit your library. Perhaps you could borrow from a friend. (You may even find this sparks a common interest where you talk, *with enthusiasm*, about what you are each planning for tea!) Alternatively, there are many gorgeous foodie magazines or websites which can be just as inspiring.

In doing this, you can turn a basic requirement - to eat or feed - into one of life's pleasures. You're bringing the joy of food back into your life. And then, when your tribe have happily devoured your new creation, you can proudly add it to your repertoire!

## Love your kitchen

If you have a family, your kitchen is likely to be a food factory. Obviously it needs to be practical, but it's also worth making it an enjoyable place to be. You are going to clock up some serious hours in this room, so why not make it as pleasant as possible? Have somewhere you can play music, or a TV if you prefer. Put fresh flowers on the windowsill. Light fragrant candles. Add some comfort and warmth. This is the heart of your home.

If you are in the enviable position of planning your kitchen, or you can make improvements, dedicate as much effort and funds as possible into making it right for you. If funds allow, opt for the surfaces that you love the most - you're going to get very familiar with wiping them! If there's room, plan for a cosy chair, even a sofa. Include inviting furniture and accessories that say your kitchen is a nice place to spend time.

View your kitchen in a more positive light. If you are going to spend a good portion of your life in there, make the best of it. This will be a far healthier and more enjoyable approach than viewing your kitchen as a place of hard labour that you can't wait to escape from. So, go now and see if there's anything you can do to make it better *for you*. Get comfortable with the idea of spending time there.

Go on, make friends with your kitchen.

## The way to their hearts

How do we seduce a love interest? How do we nurture our loved ones? How do we celebrate the great occasions of life?

There's usually food and drink involved. Food is so much more than a means of survival. It is symbolic of our love of life. The serving of food to friends and family is an important feature of many cultures. It is a chance for human interaction and bonding. It has long been associated with expressions of fondness and feeling. It is, or at least it can be, an act of love.

When you view the preparation of a meal as an act of love, it takes on a whole new dimension. Instead of just going through the motions of getting something edible on the table, it becomes an expression of what's in your heart. This is not only good for those on the receiving end, it's also hugely beneficial to the giver.

This is not to say, however, that to prove your love, every meal must be a banquet. That would soon become exhausting, and possibly lead to resentment. More important than the food you provide is the spirit in which you provide it. The description 'lovingly prepared' is perhaps the ultimate ingredient of good food.

Your love for your family can be a powerful motivating force - so why not tap into that? When you are called upon to feed others, remind yourself what you're doing - you are nurturing the ones you love. If you are responsible for the meals in your house and it's a chore that has lost its sparkle - use your feelings towards your family to inspire what and how you to feed them.

So the next time you need a good reason to venture into the kitchen, imagine that your efforts will be a demonstration of your devotion to your family.

Because, in reality, it is.

## Little mouths

If the Others in your family are able to fend for themselves, the pressure on you is somewhat diminished. Any nutrition they receive from your efforts will be a bonus, but there comes a time when their diet (and subsequent health) is in their hands.

However, if you're responsible for feeding small children, your efforts have much more impact. If we are what we eat, it follows that those we feed will be *whatever we feed them*. This is quite a responsibility. But instead of feeling over-awed by the enormity of this, why not use your innate sense of duty to your children to stimulate the energy you need to provide for them.

> If you can't feed a hundred people, then feed just one.
>
> Mother Teresa

There are days when the last thing I feel like doing is cooking a healthy meal. Yet I feel a strong, moral obligation to meet the nutritional needs of my children. For me, being a parent involves not just feeding my offspring, but feeding them *well*. So, I dig deep into my commitment to my children and haul myself into the kitchen. In fact, being committed makes it easier. There is less wondering whether I can be bothered. I know it needs to be done and this helps motivate me to get on with it. Besides, I know (from past experience) that the energy required to prepare a decent meal will pale in comparison to the guilt I will feel if I don't.

Having said that, ensuring your children are well fed needn't always be so hands on, or at least not by your hands. You will be doing yourself and your children a favour if you regularly seek or accept help. Perhaps a grandparent could give them tea once a week? Or maybe Daddy and children would enjoy a weekly homemade pizza night, where they do some bonding in the kitchen (and give you a well-earned break)?

Enlisting help is particularly advisable during the challenging phase of weaning. It's ironic that the time when you have the most influence on a child's health and future relationship with food is possibly the most frazzled period of parenting. Feeding children can be a challenge at any stage, but this one takes the teething-biscuit. Remember, then, on those days when you're all weaned-out - help is out there!

These days, *quality* baby food is readily available, prepared by experts who care almost as much about your child's nutrition as you do. These are often developed by mums who have been through this stage, who know how hard it is, and want to provide a no-compromise solution. There is no shame in succumbing to assistance during what is a particularly testing time. Better that your children have bought-in food and a happy mother, than only the finest home-cooked ingredients served up by an exhausted wreck!

As vital as nutrition is for young children, I believe even more important is a sane and healthy mother. So if there are occasions when preparing a meal is one step too far, then give yourself a break. Children are resilient creatures. If they are fed well most of the time, the odd veg-free meal isn't going to be disastrous. Many dietitians suggest an 80/20 rule, i.e., good food 80% of the time. That means there's a 20% window for giving you a break!

Also, it can be a great comfort to know that this intense period won't last forever. There will come a time when the culinary demands on you will ease up. Your children will grow and they'll increasingly eat elsewhere. Perhaps your child will become a budding chef and take over the family meals! Over the course of your lifetime, feeding children will only occupy a relatively small number of years (though it may feel like longer!). So when you next need a little encouragement, it may help to remember that this busy time, when it's always down to you, will one day be a distant memory.

And when that day comes, you'll reflect much more happily if you give it your best shot now.

## And finally...

If you find that mealtimes in your home are a big deal, you could be right. You may be going through the phase in your life when you seem to spend every waking moment preparing food, feeding others or dealing with the aftermath. Simply recognising that this is just a phase can bring some relief.

However, desperate times call for desperate measures. Given that you're dealing with a particularly demanding period, you can be forgiven for implementing some emergency tactics. In other words, build into your regime *regular time off.*

Time to get creative. There are a number of ways you can ensure a break from the kitchen without your family suffering.

For example, you may decide to eat out once a week. This need not be expensive. Perhaps you have a picnic in the park. Or you may have a regular take-away night. Even top chefs enjoy the odd take-away meal. Used as an occasional break, rather than a routine diet, it's unlikely to do much harm to your health goals.

Another option is to feed someone else's children. It doesn't take much more effort to double up on the children's tea - but you will certainly enjoy the time off when the other parent returns the favour and feeds your child!

You can even employ your charges in the production of their own tea. If you're struggling to get the food on the table whilst entertaining the children, kill two birds with one stone. Get them involved - put them to work! Most children love to help with the cooking and, amazingly, they quite like the washing-up afterwards. (Though this tends to diminish as they get older...) Plus, children are far more likely to eat what they've had a hand in preparing. You will also be teaching them valuable life lessons in relation to food and caring for others. This will help them develop an appreciation for what you do for them *every day.*

Whatever strategies work for you, try to incorporate them *regularly.* Plan ahead for intervals to the constant pressure on you to prepare endless meals. Doing this in advance will reduce those flash-points when it all suddenly becomes too much. What you're doing is quite a challenge - you are bound to need the odd break. Making sure you regularly get time off and time out of the kitchen, will make your current culinary commitments a good deal easier to stomach.

# Guilt Trip Detour

Guilt is an unproductive and insidiously harmful, negative emotion. It's bad for your health, your self-esteem and your relationships. I would never advocate using such a destructive device for any means, let alone simply getting more housework done. However, what I will suggest as a powerful motivating force is the *avoidance* of guilt.

Guilt is not just a result of doing the wrong thing. It can be a result of not doing the right thing. When you avoid what you know you ought to do, the thought of it stalks you, it lingers in the back of your mind. It can even prevent you enjoying what you put it off to do! Yet there is a staggeringly simple way of avoiding all this wailing and gnashing of teeth - just doing what should be done!

Of course, we don't really want to, which is why we avoid it in the first place. But depending how prone you are to feelings of guilt (and women are notoriously susceptible), it may actually be the easiest option in the long run. When you bear this in mind, it becomes easier to opt for long-term peace of mind in return for a little short-term effort. Recognising the unpleasant feelings that will arise from the inevitable guilt trip can be quite an effective deterrent.

*Guilt is anger directed at ourselves.*

*Peter McWilliams*

So, the next time you plan to evade that job - you know the one, the one you really ought to do - weigh up the true cost of avoiding it. In escaping the job (temporarily) you don't get off scot-free. There is a price to pay. You pay with peace of mind.

What is true in economics, also applies in the home - when you pay upfront, it always costs you less.

# Picture this...

This is an extraordinarily powerful technique that will provide motivation for your chores *and* relieve your frustration. Sound too good to be true?

Welcome to the awesome power of visualisation.

A favourite tool of Olympic athletes and great orators, visualisation harnesses the incredible power of your imagination to get the results you want. Imagination has been cited by many as the ultimate creative power. Imagination is responsible for many of humanity's greatest achievements - air travel, electricity, personal computers - all of which began as an image or vision in someone's mind. People have even claimed to have cured their ills simply by imagining good health. Einstein went as far as to say that imagination is more important than knowledge.

When you use your imagination in your domestic life, you will be astounded, not only by the end result, but also with how relatively easily you get there. So, how exactly do we make use of this powerful tool to assist with the daily grind?

Well, firstly, consider how you approach a particular loathsome task. Which part of the process do you think about? You probably direct all your attention to the actual process of the job, i.e., focussing on the work, the effort - the bit you don't like! In doing this, you conjure up in your mind all the unpleasant aspects and imagery. No wonder you don't want to do it!

Now ask yourself, why are you doing the job? The answer is because you want the result. You wash-up because you want a tidy kitchen (or you need plates!). You do the laundry because you want your family to be well-dressed. You change the beds because you don't want to be eaten alive by bedbugs. And so on...

So, instead of dwelling on the chore itself, sighing and scowling your way through it, why not focus on the *result* of the chore? Visualise the outcome. Picture that spotless sink. Smell that clean laundry. Feel those clean sheets. Focus on the whole point of the exercise - think about the best bit!

Having a vision or sense of your desired result is a powerful motivator. But when you imagine the *feelings* you will experience, you supercharge the whole process. So, try to envision the satisfaction, the sense of achievement, the enjoyment. Smile and feel proud of your efforts. Go for every sensation - touch, see, smell, taste, hear. Mentally, get into that good place where you are enjoying the results.

When you visualise the results of your efforts, you unleash the powerful driving force of your subconscious mind. You're setting a target and your brain becomes a success-seeking missile. Maxwell Maltz (author of *Psycho-cybernetics*) calls the imagination 'the ignition key to your Automatic Success Mechanism'. When you spark this process, your mind will work ceaselessly to close the gap between your vision and your reality. This will *automatically* motivate you do what is necessary to achieve your aim. Holding a mental image of the outcome serves to literally propel you towards it.

> Imagination is everything. It is the preview of life's coming attractions.
>
> Albert Einstein

So the next time you despair at the prospect of doing a job, pause, close your eyes, and turn your focus to the result. Just imagining the feeling of having finished that job will create an internal shift. You move from energy-sapping negativity to success-orientated positivity and optimism.

Ignite your imagination. Start your visual engines and set off on the road to domestic mastery. After all, if this technique can work wonders in the Olympic arena and on the world stage - surely it can make light work of a little housekeeping?

## Cheat sheets

Your imagination is like a muscle - it improves with use. But if you really find it a struggle to see the images in your mind, you may find it helpful, at first, to use a physical picture.

So the next time your house looks good (maybe when you are expecting visitors...) - take photos! This may sound extreme, but images are rapid brain-trainers. If you put these photos where you will see them, they act as constant visual reminders of what you'd like to achieve. Pictures work on a subliminal level, reinforcing your subconscious mind which will, *subconsciously*, lead you to recreate those images.

There's an added bonus in doing this. When you see a picture of your home, it almost always makes you view it slightly differently -

and you may be surprised at how nice it looks! You will actually *see* it, rather than just be aware of it. (Viewing your room through a mirror has the same effect - try it, it's fun!) Familiar images soon become uninteresting to the brain, so you stop seeing your home as a newcomer would. By taking photos of your home, you get to see it from a new angle, which just might endear you more to where you live.

Alternatively, if you can't wait for your home to have a good day (or it never has a good day!) grab some interiors magazines. Find a picture that makes you say, *I want my kitchen/bedroom/bathroom to look like that!* Then tear out the page and stick it on your fridge or dressing table or bathroom mirror.

In this way, you are training your brain to see a beautiful home as the norm. Your mind becomes focused on the results rather than on the efforts. So when it's time to do the work involved, your mind can readily see the point and purpose, which results in more motivation and less wearying resentment.

If you're in any doubt as to the effectiveness of this technique, I could direct you to numerous resources on the power of imagination. (I found *Directing the Movies of Your Mind* audiobook to be a good introduction.) But the most potent argument will always be your own evidence - so try it! What harm can it do? And once you discover this latent power, you can apply it to all areas of your life, from money matters to marital or parenting issues. I guarantee you'll be amazed by the results.

So if you need some encouragement to get going on your chores - flood your mind with images of your desired outcome. Focus on the ultimate reason for doing the jobs. Then picture how good you'll feel when the necessary jobs are done.

And before you know it - they will be.

> By believing passionately in something that does not yet exist, we create it.
>
> Nikos Kazantzakis

# It's a love thing

Love begins by taking care
of the closest ones -
the ones at home.

*Mother Teresa*

What is housework, if not an expression of love?

Housework is essentially care-work. The domestic routine is largely the maintenance of your family's basic needs - food, clothing, shelter, etc. Assuming you love your family, love is probably the reason you take on this work. Why else would you provide such a service without payment or reward?

It's very easy to lose sight of this, though. As we become so absorbed in what needs to be done, we may forget the original reason for doing it. Lost in the mundane details, we fail to see the bigger picture - that a family is a wonderful thing! This is understandable, given the constant and repetitive nature of much of domestic work. How ever much we may love our families, without the right mindset, Housework Blues can sometimes get a hold.

So it can be helpful to remember what, or rather who, you're doing this for - and why. Remind yourself that you take care *of* them because you care *about* them. When you go back to basics, it's a love thing.

Love is the reason we have this work to do. It's our innate quest for love that propels us to create families in the first place. So love has quite a bit to answer for! Helpfully, though, love also equips us with the means to do the work.

Love is a compelling emotion. It makes us want to do nice things for those we love. Love makes us want to give - of our time, our money, ourselves. People have even given their lives in the name of love. Can you think of a stronger motivating force? So, if you feel love for your family, that is an incredible source of power that *you can tap into*.

I think that's worth repeating: your love for your family is a source of power that you can tap into.

Simply summoning your feelings for your family can be a powerful motivator in taking care of them. Recognising the love you feel for them can make you *naturally inclined* to do things for them. After all, when we love someone, not only are we prepared to do what makes them happy, we actually *want* to do it. Voluntarily. Even joyfully! When we feel love, we're inspired to express it. We have a strong desire to let those we love know about it. We also tend to do more than is required, more than the bare minimum. And best of all, we do this in a spirit of joy and giving - which has got to be more fun than a spirit of begrudging resentment.

So, by tapping into your feelings of devotion, not only will you be more productive, you will be happier about it. And when you actually *intend* your work as an expression of love, far from being subservient, you become empowered. You are harnessing one of the most powerful driving forces on the planet.

But the perks don't stop there. When you express your love, it's not just the object of your affection that benefits. Showing you care actually makes *you* feel good. We are so built that even the selfless aspects of love, giving, sacrifice, etc are rewarding *to us*. When we love, we're naturally motivated to give because we find pleasure in doing so.

However... the trouble comes when this natural tendency is obscured by feelings of resentment or injustice or frustration. In other words, our 'issues'. But such is the power of love that merely focusing on it can obliterate these negative emotions. It's impossible to focus on two things at the same time, so if your mind is firmly on the love stuff, there's less room for any irritation.

> I like hugs and
> I like kisses.
> But what I really
> love is help
> with the dishes!
>
> *Unknown*

Within the home, keeping love front and centre will help to ease your burden of care and reduce resentment. This is not to suggest that the only way for a woman to express her love is through housework. Obviously, there are more ways to express our love than via mundane domestic maintenance. But it is *one way* that any person (regardless of gender) can express their affection.

Neither am I suggesting that a messy house indicates a lack of love. There are many sage proverbs that recommend putting quality family time before housework. My point is merely to highlight the *potential* for transforming repetitive boring chores into a demonstration of love. Taking care of your family *can be* an additional way of expressing your feelings towards them, relieving much of your angst in the process.

Of course, you do need to be realistic. Whilst it's true that simple acts of care and maintenance can say 'I love you' far more powerfully than spoken words, there may be days when you feel everyone is oblivious to your efforts. The cruel irony of housework is that people only tend to notice when it's *not* done. People don't appreciate the laundering of their socks until the sock drawer is bare.

But even if they don't or can't vocalise it, they will have a sense of feeling cared for, even if only on a subconscious level. And if you love them, don't you want to meet their basic human need of being nurtured? So accept that they're unlikely to acknowledge every single thing you do for them. (But then, think of the person who raised you - did you thank them for every act of caring? Did you even notice?) Also, you may never know which particular acts have touched their hearts. But when you spend a good deal of your time and energy in lovingly tending to your family, you can be sure that in some small, ordinary way - they will inevitably feel it.

Choosing to view our work as an expression of our love - *work we have to do anyway* - is a win-win-win solution. You get to express your love, adding a sense of value to your work. Your family feel more loved and cared for (and may, as a result, love you even more!) Plus your home will undoubtedly feel the benefit - any home that is kept in a spirit of loving kindness is bound to be good feng shui!

When you imbue your domestic work with your love for your family, it transports the mundane into an act of devotion. In those small acts of taking care of your family, you reflect your dedication to them. This gives purpose and meaning to keeping a home.

That's some power. It's the power of love.

## Love supplies

It can be tricky to love someone, warts and all.

When you live with someone, there are going to be things they do that annoy you. Having perfectly behaved housemates is not a realistic option. Just because you want to share your home and your life with someone does not mean their ways will automatically be in sync with yours.

Albert Einstein once quipped, 'Women marry men hoping they will change. Men marry women hoping they will not. Each is inevitably disappointed.' Our sex is notorious for trying to 'tweak' others to meet our expectations. But is that really what love is all about?

This is where the more testing aspects of love kick in - acceptance and forgiveness. You may be unable to control the way your loved ones like to live, but you do get to decide how you react to their little foibles. And if you love them, a degree of acceptance is required. Success guru Brian Tracy goes as far as to say, 'The greatest gift that you can give to others is the gift of unconditional love and acceptance.' Whilst motivational speaker Wayne Dyer cites 'the quiet acceptance of what is' as his definition of enlightenment.

Striving for acceptance in your home will not only be a great gift to your family, it will benefit you as well. And it may help you to remember there's something in it for you, because it's not always going to be easy...

In fact, the notion of acceptance can really test your feelings for your loved ones. You may tell your family that you love them every day, but that's the relatively easy part. The true test comes when you are asked to prove it. To accept them when they do that thing that really bugs you - even though you've asked them *repeatedly* not to do it! - you'll need to draw on your supplies of love. But then, that's what it's there for!

> Love begins at home, and it is not how much we do... but how much love we put in that action.
>
> *Mother Teresa*

After all, didn't you select to have these significant others in your life? Love is the reason you have their 'stuff' to deal with. It may involve more work for you (in the case of children, it will definitely involve more work for you), but that's part of the deal of having them in your life. That's just the way it is, so you will save yourself much heartache if you can manage to accept it.

A natural spin-off from acceptance is forgiveness. When you take people as they are, not how you want them to be, you automatically become more forgiving. This has one tremendous advantage for you - less anger!

Again, forgiveness may take some work but if you can manage it, the payoff is worthwhile. Forgiveness is powerful and there are some great books devoted solely to the amazing results that stem from a forgiving attitude. The Sedona Method is based on this principle of forgiveness and it claims to be the key to your lasting happiness, success, peace and emotional well-being. How would you like those results?

★

So, in your pursuit of domestic bliss, why not harness the amazing power of love and strive for a little more acceptance and forgiveness? Draw on your reserves of this powerful emotion to bring more peace to your heart and more harmony to your home. Love can both motivate you and ease your struggle. You'll also find that, the more often love is the driving force in your domestic schedule, the more love you'll feel in your home. You will love your life and your family more. You'll undoubtedly love yourself more. You may even learn to love your chores (sounds unlikely, I know - but some people do.).

Don't underestimate the power of love in your home. If this stuff can make the world go round, surely it can assist with a bit of housework.

# Charity begins at home

John Assaraf, (author of *Having It All*), claims that *contribution* is one of the highest functions of human need. He says, 'We *want* to contribute. It makes us feel good about what we are, who we are. It gives us purpose and meaning.'

We have an innate desire to give and share, to help and care for our fellow human beings. You probably already contribute to society in some way - perhaps you donate your money to charity or volunteer your time for a worthy cause. As a race, we somehow know that this is a right and good way to live, to not be totally self-serving but to do our bit for others.

The most conventional way to contribute is to give to those in great need. Whilst this is a generous and rewarding act, it's not the only way we can give. If we feel an in-built sense to reach out and care for others, could we not also direct this spirit of generosity a little closer to home?

Isn't it just as valid to give freely to our family as it is to donate to a cause half-way round the world? If it's right that you give of yourself for the benefit of others - what about doing that within the walls of your own home?

> It is when you give of yourself that you truly give.
>
> *Kahlil Gibran*

You may argue that your family aren't in great need. Whilst, hopefully, that's true, Mother Teresa said that, more than food, humans need love. Your family are human beings who need to feel cared for and loved. They need nurturing and attention. You can make a difference in the world simply by the way you treat the people in your home.

Yet we often tend to give more generously to perfect strangers. Why is this? Perhaps we suspect that if we serve those close to us, they'll take advantage, abuse our generosity, not appreciate us? But surely, the point of a charitable act is what you *give*, not what you get in return. Otherwise it's not charity, it's trade.

Keeping a home, raising a family, nurturing a supportive environment, these are good works. By doing these things, with a willing heart, you are most certainly doing your bit. Viewing your domestic work as an act of contribution (something you are innately driven to perform) can help to inspire you on those days when the Housework Blues are looming. Though it seems illogical, by giving more freely, with no expectation of a return, you will find your work and your life much more rewarding.

Plus, looking upon your duties not as mundane chores but as opportunities for charitable acts, will be good for you - good for your heart, your soul and your peace of mind. And since the way we care for our families can, and will, make a difference in the world, this charity may begin at home, but the ripple effects of our kindness will travel much, much further.

> Every charitable act is a stepping stone towards heaven.
>
> *Henry Ward Beecher*

# Love where you live

Hopefully, by this point, you have discovered many valid and compelling reasons to tackle your housework. If I've done my job well, you'll now see how taking care of your home can benefit your relationships, your health, your career, your finances, your self-esteem, your time, your peace of mind, your goals, your sanity, your well-being, your families, your soul, your ego and your happiness.

Though it was probably your negative feelings towards your home that drew you to this book in the first place, it's my hope that, already, you're beginning to view your home in a new, more positive light. But in case you have any lingering frustrations or resentments in the maintenance of your abode, it may help to reflect on just how much your home means to you.

Perhaps the most over-worked cliché says it best - it's where our heart is. It's the place we can call our own. It's where we go to retreat from a frenzied or frightening world. Home is the place we can freely reveal who we truly are. It's a reflection of our personalities, an expression of our souls. Home is where we raise our families and nurture our relationships. It's where we invite our friends and loved ones to share in our celebrations and achievements.

> A house is made
> of walls and beams;
> a home is built
> with love and dreams.
>
> *Unknown*

It's the backdrop for so many of our memories. It's a place to rest, relax, feel comforted and safe. When we're world weary or weather-beaten, there's nothing quite like the feeling of coming home.

This place, however so humble, has a unique role in our lives and an unparalleled place in our hearts.

Home is far more than just a roof over our heads. Its role goes way beyond mere protection from the elements. It affects how we feel and how we think about ourselves. It has the potential to hold a powerful, even magical influence over our whole life - even when we're not there.

Our home is not just significant in our success and happiness - it's vital. In her beautiful book *Space Matters*, Kathleen Cox endorses what she calls our sublimely critical space. 'Home should celebrate who we are and what we love. Home ought to serve us well, make us feel good and protect the core of our essence - our soul.'

Recognising the incredible role our home plays in our lives highlights just how much is at stake in the care - or neglect - of where we live. When we reconnect to the value of our home, when we realise the extent of its effect on our lives, we naturally become more respectful and appreciative of our little corner of the world. When we stop seeing the home purely as a place of chores and maintenance, there's a chance to treasure it as the wonderful sanctuary it's meant to be.

In this light, the upkeep of a home is less oppressive. It becomes a labour of love. There is undoubtedly work involved in having a home, but in the same way that children and families involves a degree of work - the payoff makes it all worthwhile. Home offers us much in return. We reap rich dividends for our labours. Our efforts are always rewarded, one way or another.

Admittedly, there are times when the upkeep seems endless, futile, repetitive, monotonous and mundane. But remember there is real value in this work. Though it may be unpaid, unacknowledged, even unnoticed, the gains of taking care of your home are priceless. The returns are your quality of life.

One of the biggest frustrations of the domestic realm is that, in doing housework, we're missing out on something else, something better or more important. But isn't it true that we will miss out on far more by neglecting our homes? If we don't take care of it, how well will it take care of us?

*To be happy at home is the result of all ambition.*

*Samuel Johnson*

I leave you with this challenge. Go now and rediscover your home. Reflect on exactly what it means to you and the crucial role it plays in your life. See if, deep down, you love where you live. And if you find that you don't - could you learn to? Put the heart back in hearth. Put some love back in your home.

Dorothy was right: there is no place like it.

293

# Outro

## Over to you!

So, you have reached the end of this book. Hopefully, though, this will just be the beginning of a new, happier phase in your domestic life.

You are now armed to the hilt with coping strategies, enlightened ideas, supportive beliefs, positive affirmations and helpful insights. All that's left is for you to take these ideas into the field, to view your challenges in a new light and find happier solutions.

My hope is that already, you will have shifted from a sense of fury, frustration or despair to a calmer, more optimistic mindset. Of course, a bonus side effect would be more efficiency and competence in your domestic role. But more important than being the perfect homemaker is your sanity and your peace of mind.

The sole aim of this book has been to soothe the angst within. And with this in mind, I offer one final word of advice:

## Keep calm...

There is no need to put all these ideas into practice immediately. It took me close to two years to implement most of these changes - some of which I'm still working on.

Be patient with yourself and your results. It may take time. After all, you're working on habits and beliefs built up over a lifetime. Sometimes improvements may be like a thunderbolt, but more often they're far more subtle. Either way is progress.

## ...and carry on.

Don't give up. Remember, there are no failures, only feedback. So go easy on yourself. Surviving Housework Blues will be more of a journey than a destination. But if you've taken on board the ideas in this book, you cannot fail to make progress in the right direction - the direction of a calmer and happier you.

Wishing you health, happiness and harmony within your home,

*Danielle*

P.S. As and when you do find more peace with your housework - I would dearly love to hear about it. So feel free to email me at: danielle@houseworkblues.com

I look forward to reading your success stories!

# About the author

Throughout this book, you may have wondered about the author's home. Is it kept spotless? Is her family harmonious? Is her mental health exemplary?

In other words, do I practice what I preach?

Well, the only answer I can give you, in all honesty is: I try. But much as I aspire to the perfect home life, I am realistic. I have a family and though they are wonderful and talented in many ways - they are what I lovingly refer to as Messy Ones. And though I'm trying to encourage them to see the advantages of organisation and independent maintenance - I still have a long way to go.

However, the habits of my family or indeed the state of my home are not what this book is about. I wrote this book to document the changes that had occurred within my heart and mind. My homemaking skills may have vastly improved in recent months, but the most outstanding result has been to the changes to my attitude.

I am more calm and accepting. I am less angry and stressed. I am infinitely happier with my little lot. Though my workload hasn't altered much – I've learned to simultaneously manage more and fret less. So my home is a nicer place to be and I'm less likely to explode at the slightest abandoned sock. For me, that's success.

Though, I still don't adore the domestic stuff, I have come to terms with it. I no longer fight and resent it. I am, in short, surviving my Housework Blues. I may even have conquered some for good. And I believe these are the only qualifications necessary to write this book.

But not only did I feel I could write this book - I also passionately believed that I *should* write it. Since I am living proof that it's possible to make peace with the surprisingly common domestic demons, I felt duty-bound to share these solutions with women everywhere. Because if I can do it, they can too. And I feel certain that our world will be a slightly nicer place when they do.

So, in answer to your ponderings: I have reached a calmer karma within my home and I'm looking forward to further improvements.

I wish this and more for you.

# Suggested reading

Throughout this book, I've included details of books and websites which develop the discussed ideas more deeply. However, there are a few resources that I would recommend to everybody (and regularly do!) The material in these books has undoubtedly changed the course of my life for the better and may well do the same for you.

As always, let your famous intuition guide you as to which ones hold the answer for you.

Enjoy!

★ *Don't Sweat the Small Stuff* - Richard Carlson

★ *The Success Principles* - Jack Canfield

★ *Having It All* - John Assaraf

★ *Psycho-Cybernetics* - Dr Maxwell Maltz

★ *Secrets of the Millionaire Mind* - T Harv Eker

★ *The Cleaning Bible* - Kim and Aggie

★ *The Secret* - Rhonda Byrne (Audiobook)

★ *Quantum NLP* - Christiane Turner (Audiobook)

★ *Goals* - Brian Tracy (Audiobook)

★ *It's not about the money* - Bob Proctor (Audiobook)

★ *Mood Mapping* - Dr Liz Miller

★ *How to Be Brilliant* - Michael Hepple

★ *Creating Affluence* - Deepak Chopra (Audiobook)

★ *The Seven Spiritual Laws of Success* - Deepak Chopra (Audiobook)

## Resources

For a regularly updated list of further reading and relevant resources, please visit www.houseworkblues.com. Here you'll find news, reviews and useful views to help you tackle your Housework Blues.

See you there!

Lightning Source UK Ltd.
Milton Keynes UK
15 January 2011
165771UK00001B/29/P